613.7
S85y4

teach ®
yourself

yoga

JAN 06

DEC 09

AUG -7 2005

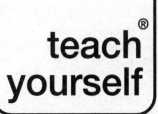

yoga

mary stewart

The **teach yourself** series does
exactly what it says, and it works.
For over 60 years, more than
40 million people have learnt over
750 subjects the **teach yourself**
way, with impressive results.

be where you want to be
with **teach yourself**

For UK order queries: please contact Bookpoint Ltd, 130 Milton Park, Abingdon, Oxon OX14 4SB. Telephone: +44 (0)1235 827720. Fax: +44 (0)1235 400454. Lines are open from 9.00–18.00, Monday to Saturday, with a 24-hour message answering service. You can also order through our website www.madabout books.com.

For USA order queries: please contact McGraw-Hill Customer Services, PO Box 545, Blacklick, OH 43004-0545, USA. Telephone: 1-800-722-4726. Fax: 1-614-755-5645.

For Canada order queries: please contact McGraw-Hill Ryerson Ltd, 300 Water St, Whitby, Ontario L1N 9B6, Canada. Telephone: 905 430 5000. Fax: 905 430 5020.

Long-renowned as the authoritative source for self-guided learning – with more than 30 million copies sold worldwide – the *Teach Yourself* series includes over 300 titles in the fields of languages, crafts, hobbies, business and education.

British Library Cataloguing in Publication Data
A catalogue record for this title is available from The British Library.

Library of Congress Catalog Card Number: On file

First published in UK 1998 by Hodder Headline Ltd., 338 Euston Road, London, NW1 3BH.

First published in US 1998 by Contemporary Books, a Division of The McGraw-Hill Companies, 1 Prudential Plaza, 130 East Randolph Street, Chicago, IL 60601 USA.

The 'Teach Yourself' name and logo are registered trade marks of Hodder & Stoughton Ltd.

This edition published 2003

Copyright © 1998, 2003 Mary Stewart

Typeset by Transet Limited, Coventry, England.
Printed in Great Britain for Hodder & Stoughton Educational, a division of Hodder Headline Ltd, 338 Euston Road, London NW1 3BH by Cox & Wyman Ltd, Reading, Berkshire.

Impression number   7 6 5 4 3 2 1
Year   2009 2008 2007 2006 2005 2004
                    2003

contents

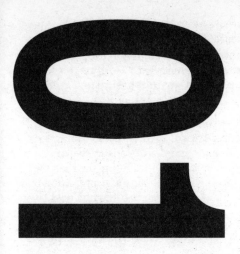

01

what is Yoga?

In this chapter you will learn:
- the history of Yoga
- the origins of Indian philosophy
- the eight steps of classical Yoga
- Hatha Yoga and Tantra.

Yoga originated in the subcontinent of India thousands of years ago and during its long history has taken many different forms. The word Yoga means concentration or contemplation and can be translated as 'union'. It means Union with God, of the soul with the Divine, and also a practical way of physical and ethical discipline and meditation that is focused on that goal.

Yoga has been defined as 'the stilling of the restless fluctuations of the mind' (*Yoga Sutras* book 1 verse 2). It is the searching for freedom from the world of images and distortions in which our thinking is trapped through fear and conditioning, so that we can recognize the Spirit of God within us. This concept, known to all major religions as humankind's search for wholeness, is universal. For those who believe that we are caught in a continuous round of births, deaths and rebirths, each life patterned on the actions of past lives, Yoga is also a way of freedom from the cycle of reincarnation. This idea of the residue of our former lives colouring the present, where we have a chance to redress the balance, is the doctrine of Karma.

Yoga addresses all aspects of our lives from muscles and joints to tendencies buried deep in our subconscious, and through practice we have a chance to work through our negative tendencies rendering them inoperative in the future and so gaining liberation.

The ancient teaching of Yoga does not separate the body from the mind and the path of Yoga always included bodily posture and breathing as an important part of the practice of concentration. Both the Sanskrit scriptures, the *Upanishads*, written about 600 BC, and the *Bhagavad Gita*, dating some 200 years later, advise 'sitting with the body, head and neck erect' when you meditate. The Yoga Sutras list both posture (Asana) and breath control (Pranayama) among the Eight Steps of Yoga. This emphasis on bodily posture and breathing is the aspect of Yoga that is best known outside India. Indeed for many people it is all they know of Yoga. To use the body in a religious sense is an alien concept for many of us, for most religious people tend to deal with their physical self by disciplines such as fasting to subdue the flesh, and think of attention to the body as a dangerous self-indulgence rather than a pathway for grace.

Yoga is as old as civilization. Its first traces were found in the prehistoric ruins of the Indus Valley in what is now Pakistan. Here carved seals were discovered, some of which showed a figure seated in a Yoga position which is still practised today.

The script used by these Indus Valley people has not yet been deciphered but from their well planned cities and buildings we know that theirs was an advanced culture pre-dating the migration of the Aryans into India from the north.

The earliest written references to Yoga are in the *Vedas* (2500–600 BC). Written in Sanskrit they are the hymns of the Aryan people, the *Rg Veda* is the oldest Indo-European philosophical text, and the *Vedas* are the roots of the later philosophies and religious practices of India. The later Vedas, known as *Upanishads*, differed from the nature worship and rituals of the earlier hymns.

'Upanishad' literally translates as 'sitting next to' and they seem to be written from the depth of personal experience as if from a Teacher – Guru to disciples. This handing down of knowledge from Teacher to pupil is the traditional way that Yoga has been passed down for thousands of years, right up to the present day. It explains the widely differing ways of following the path.

The *Vedas* are hymns to the outer world of creation, the writers of the *Upanishads* spoke of the inner search of the mystic for direct experience of the Divine and of the philosopher's search for understanding.

The *Upanishads* contain ideas which are still part of Yoga practice today. The *Katha* Upanishad describes the Eternal Self – Atman riding in a chariot which is the body, the intellect – Buddhi is the driver and the mind the reins. The Senses are the horses. This Upanishad tells us that the Atman cannot be experienced through learning or reason but only through direct realization or insight: 'Where the five senses and the mind are still, and reason itself rests in Silence then begins the Path Supreme'; and 'This is Yoga … the beginning and the end.'

The *Mandukya* Upanishad gives the theory of the four states of consciousness, which are waking, dreaming, deep sleep and a fourth state turiya, which is reality. It relates these states to the mystic syllable OM. In Sanskrit O is a dipthong of A and U and the syllable is analyzed as:

A – the waking state,
U – dreaming,
M – deep sleep, and

the whole sound as alone being reality.

The *Tattiriya* Upanishad contains the teaching of the five sheaths of the body and the five vital breaths that pervade it.

The *Maitri* Upanishad, foreshadowing Patanjali's classical Path, advocates a sixfold Yoga of restraint of breath, withdrawal of the senses, meditation, concentration, contemplation and absorption.

The *Bhagavad Gita*, which was written about 600 BC, came at the end of the Vedic period. It is inserted into the epic story of the *Mahabarata* and contains a poetic revelation of Yogic teaching. The *Mahabarata* tells the story of two warring factions of a royal family. At the decisive battle, the archer prince Arjuna hesitates as he is unwilling to kill his friends and family who oppose him. Arjuna's chariot is driven by the God, Krishna, who in the role of Teacher explains to Arjuna the Yoga of Selfless Action (Karma Yoga), of Knowledge (Jnana Yoga) and of Adoration (Bhakti Yoga). The Yoga of the *Gita* is love, the paths of action, knowledge and adoration are complementary.

> Spiritual experience is above the Scriptures. (*Bhagavad Gita*, 2 vv 52 & 3)
>
> only through the renunciation of the fruits of action is there Freedom. (*Bhagavad Gita*, 4)
>
> Only by love can men see me and know me and come to me. (*Bhagavad Gita*, 11 v 54)

The *Bhagavad Gita* was written at a time of flowering of philosophical and religious thought. The orthodox systems of Hinduism developed, as did Jainism. In Judaism the prophesies of Isaiah were written and Gautama, the Buddha (the Enlightened One), lived and taught.

The Buddha was born around 568 BC, the son of a king from the borders of India and Nepal. When he was 30 years old he left his father's palace, his life of luxury and his family, to wander for six years in search of enlightenment through the practice of Yoga. Finally seated under a tree he attained his goal and for the rest of his life he taught his followers the way to freedom. Buddhism, which rejected the caste system and the authority of the *Vedas*, developed separately from Hinduism and eventually virtually died out in India while spreading elsewhere in Asia. Yoga practices, which were absorbed into Buddhist teaching, were thus carried into such countries as Tibet, Sri Lanka, Thailand, Korea, Indonesia and China.

The Six Systems

The rise of Buddhism and Jainism meant that the more conservative thinkers remaining within the teaching of the *Vedas* had to defend their beliefs, and adopt a more analytical way of reasoning to underpin the poetically expressed spiritual ideas of the *Upanishads*. The six orthodox systems of philosophy that resulted were set down in Darsanas.

The Darsanas developed over many years in the post-Buddhist pre-Christian era. They went through a long period of gestation, which lasted many generations, and were than crystalized in the form of Aphorisms or Sutras. The very succinctness of those Aphorisms, which would have been handed down by word of mouth, necessitated their interpretation by commentaries, which not only elucidated the teaching but defended it against its rivals. Some of the older commentaries are considered almost as important as the Aphorisms themselves.

The Darsanas were not just intellectual exercises, but knowledge that was intended as a practical guide for living. Although they were apparently isolated systems, they developed with an awareness of each other and belonged to an overall plan. The six systems are Nyaya, Vaisisika, Samkya, Yoga, Purva Mimamsa and Vedanta. The Buddha had remained silent regarding a positive reality beneath the world of change and shifting mental states. The Six Systems however affirmed an objective reality and represented the continuity of Vedic Teachings. The *Upanishads* were considered to be original enlightened wisdom – Sruti – such knowledge being unattainable by human reasoning but realized by direct intuition. These teachings, however, had covered a wide spectrum which allowed plenty of scope for interpretation.

The spiritual experiences of the *Upanishads* were subjected to logical reasoning, each system having its own doctrine and the meanings of common words sometimes differing between them. Ultimately reason was subject to intuition because the source of life is not to be understood by logic alone for, as the *Upanishads* show, there is a state that transcends intellectual knowledge.

All the systems accepted the idea of endless rhythms of world creation and dissolution spanning aeons of time and also endless cycles of birth and rebirth in which human kind was trapped through ignorance. Freedom could only come through a superconscious recognition of the truth. The truth of the eternal spirit that really is, as distinguished from the material with which we mistakenly identify. Unselfish acts and compassion, although advocated, could only lead to good lives within the cycle of rebirth; superconscious transcendence alone brought freedom.

The Samkya and Yoga systems

The Samkya gives the theory that underlies the practical discipline of yoga. In this system Purusha – Eternal Spirit (The Knower) and Prakrti – the Material Cause of the Universe (The Known) are uncreated realities. Prakrti – the Known is the basis of all created matter both physical and psychical. Prakrti is a force of three constituent tendencies, the Gunas. Rajas – activity, Tamas – inertia and Sattva – clarity. When these tendencies are in a state of equilibrium there is a state of suspension, creation begins when the balance is disturbed by the presence of consciousness and evolution begins.

The intelligence which develops through this action is not Purusha but reflects it and identifies with it. Each evolving ego possesses a physical body and a subtle psychical body, these are Prakrti, the Spirit alone is Purusha. Liberation in Samkya is attained through the practice of Yoga.

Patanjali's *Yoga Sutras* (Raja Yoga)

One of the oldest of these six systems of philosophical thought was Yoga. The systems were written down in the form of *Sutras*. Sutra means a thread, and the writings were short phrases strung together so they could be easily memorized. The *Yoga Sutras* were written by Patanjali who is thought to have lived between 200 BC and AD 200. His exact identity is uncertain as there may have been more than one person of this name writing around those dates. Yoga is extremely ancient with a long period of development prior to the collating of the *Sutras*. The *Sutras* do not refer to or refute any of the other systems or Buddhism, although the first commentaries seem to be written with knowledge of Buddhist ideas. Patanjali's *Sutras* contained the essence of what was an established practical discipline, already well known through the spreading of Buddhist teaching. Like the Buddha he wrote of an eightfold path which encompassed the whole of human behaviour, from everyday activities, posture and breathing to the freedom of self-realization through meditation. This classical Yoga system is sometimes called Raja Yoga as opposed to the more physically orientated disciplines of Hatha Yoga. The eight 'Angas' or limbs of Patanjali's path are:

1 The five universal moral commandments (Yama):

Non-violence – Ahimsa
Truth – Satya
Not stealing – Asteya
Continence – Bramacharya
Non coveting – Aparigraha

In Yoga practice the Yamas are called 'The Great Vow' as they apply universally. Many people may follow some of the rules to some extent. For example a fisherman might practise non-violence, with the exception of violence to fish, but in Yoga these rules apply in every case regardless of place, time, caste or duty.

2 The five personal disciplines (Niyama):

Purity – Saucha
Contentment – Santosa
Austerity – Tapas
Study – Svadhyaya
Devotion to God – Isvara Prandidhana

Purity implies purity of body and of the mind; contentment is the absence of desire; austerity, study and devotion to God are the prerequisites for serious Yoga practice, see page 13.

The Yamas and Niyamas also develop through the practice of the last three meditative steps: Dharana, Dhyana and Samadi. Meditation addresses the latent seeds of violence, untruth, acquisitiveness, and so on, that lie in the subconscious. Only when these are eliminated can the Yamas and Niyama be truly established. 'In the truly virtuous', says Patanjali 'their influence extends to the world around them' (*Yoga Sutras*, Ch. 2, v. 35).

3 Bodily posture (Asana)

This should be steady and relaxed say the *Sutras*. Anyone who has tried to practise meditation and sit still for any length of time will understand how difficult these simple requirements are. To sit relaxed yet upright, alert and perfectly still for just half an hour or so without getting an aching back and pins and needles in your feet is an art. The practice of 'stilling the mind' or meditation affects and is affected by the body in other ways too; mental distractions manifest themselves physically as tensions in the body, and pain and tiredness affect concentration. The purpose of the traditional Yoga postures is that the body will be able to sit straight, steady and relaxed so that the mind can be undisturbed. The steady, erect, relaxed posture needed for meditation entails a true understanding of the force of gravity that is constantly pulling us towards the centre of the earth. Through the practice of posture we develop the ability to sit, stand, move or balance in accordance with its laws, without aggression and without expending unnecessary energy.

4 Regulated breathing (Pranayama)

Understanding natural forces and the use of energy is also the concept behind the practice of Pranayama. Prana means the vital energy within us of which breath is only a part. Through breathing techniques the balance of this energy can be regulated and redirected, just as the physical body can be changed through postures. Patanjali says that knowledge of posture is essential before Pranayama can be practised.

5 Withdrawal of the senses (Pratyahara)

The practice of detachment from outside disturbance and distractions, which is a prerequisite for the following steps.

6 Concentration (Dharana)

7 Meditation (Dhyana)

8 Illumination (Samadhi)

These last three stages are known as the Inner Path – Samyama – and are explained in Chapter 6, Meditation.

Bhakti Yoga

In more detail, Bhakti Yoga is the mystical path of personal devotion and longing for God, where union with the divine is reached by sheer love alone. From the seventh century there was a series of Bhakti movements in India. An alternative to materialism, these rejected the established religion, the caste system and ritual through which a devotee could try to obtain salvation, and instead sought direct personal religious experience. These followers were from all castes and social backgrounds.

Patanjali's classical Yoga defines methods of concentration as being with object, or concentration on the formless limitless infinite. Bhakti Yoga is also said to divide those who practise Bhakti devoted to a personal accessible Saviour, usually in Hinduism Krishna or Rama, and those whose devotion is offered to an impersonal deity.

One of the most intense expressions of personal devotion can be found in the *Gita Govinda* by the twelfth century Bengali poet Jayadeva which tells of Radha's longing for Krishna. The *Vacanas* (lyrics) of the medieval Vivasaiva saints are examples of devotion to an impersonal deity. They sought the experience of God, which is a gift of grace, which is not to be obtained through good works or rituals which seek to manipulate the cosmos:

> Feed the poor
> tell the truth
> make water places
> build tanks for a town
> you may then go to heaven
> after death, but you'll get nowhere
> near the truth of our Lord.

> And the man who knows our Lord
> he gets no results.   *Allama.*

The Vacanas are monotheistic and A. K. Ramanuja says in his introduction to '*Speaking of Siva*' that 'Christian missionaries ... speculated that Bhakti attitudes were the result of early Christian influence and Christian texts and lives strike many Hindus as variants of Bhakti.'

In the Christian tradition the '*Hymns of Divine Love*' by the tenth century Byzantine mystic St Simeon the New Theologian and the poems of the sixteenth century Spanish St John of the Cross have much in common with the writings of the Bhakti saints.

Hatha Yoga

The *Hatha Yoga Pradipika*, the *Siva Samhita* and the *Gherandha Samhita* were written in the Middle Ages. These are concerned, at some length with physical exercises and breathing and cleansing techniques as a means of purifying the body to make it fit for transcendence, although the need for ethical discipline and meditation is also emphasized. Today Raja Yoga is taken to mean meditation and Hatha Yoga physical exercises. Strictly speaking this is incorrect as both the Hatha Yoga writings and Patanjali's *Sutras* contain all the elements of the eight limbs of Yoga.

Tantra – extension of understanding

Since the Aryans had migrated into the Indian subcontinent bringing with them the Vedic teachings of ritual sacrifice and a priestly caste, the pre-Aryan religion continued to be practised by wandering groups of ascetics known as Vratyas. It is probably from these pre-Aryan influences that Tantra developed in both Hinduism and Buddhism. The Tantric texts written in the first millennium AD, are symbolic and extremely obscure. There is an emphasis on secrecy and the paramount importance of initiation by a Guru. Physical exercises are seen as a direct method of gaining religious experience, the use of sound (mantra), sight (yantra or mandala), light (trataka) and the sublimation of sexual union all being used for this purpose.

In the Tantric and Hatha Yoga writings a whole physiology of a subtle body has been developed; this is said to be composed of finer forms of energy than are detectable by modern scientific investigation. According to these esoteric teachings the body consists of five layers or koshas, with only the most gross layer being realized at the physical level. Within this subtle body there lies a cosmos that mirrors the external cosmos. This revolves round the spine and contains the Sun, Moon and stars as well as the elements of earth, air, fire, water and sky. This inner universe is pervaded by the vital energy Prana, itself a composite of subsidiary energies. Prana is channelled along pathways known as nadis. There are said to be hundreds of these, the two principal ones being the pingala, which carries the solar energy HA, and the ida, which carries the lunar energy THA.

The goal of Hatha Yoga is to channel these vital energies into the central channel Susumna, which lies along the axis of the spine. This central channel is entwined by a double helix of the solar and lunar channels, the energy at its base being dormant. This dormant energy is described as being in the form of a coiled serpent (Kundalini), which blocks the lower entrance to the Susumna with her mouth as she sleeps. The aim of the practices described in the Hatha Yoga and Tantric writings is to arouse this dormant energy and drive it up the central channel to activate the centres known as Chakras (wheels or lotuses), which lie along its path, until finally the awakened creative force unites with the static force (Shiva) in the final chakra at the crown of the head. This brings about a transformation of consciousness. In these teachings the Asanas are a means of training the body to prepare it for this redistribution of energy.

The Chakras lie along the line of the spine in the subtle body and are thought to correspond to nerve plexus in the physical body. According to some interpretations of the old texts the junction between the sacrum and the fifth lumbar vertebra is the root of the Susumna where the energy is blocked. On a purely physical level, this is a point where there is mechanical stress – the other point being where the top two vertebrae articulate with the skull. When you do the Asanas these two points at the bottom and top of the mobile part of the spine should always move away from each other along the line of the spine so that the curves can elongate and straighten.

Each Asana is a therapy in itself. With the base of the pose firmly grounded through contact with the gravitational pull of the earth, the exhalation is the impetus for the spine to stretch; the elongation as you go into the pose serves to adjust and straighten the body, realigning postural deviations caused by right- or left-handedness and improving spinal problems. In esoteric terms this balances the energies of the sun HA and the moon THA and in physical terms releases stiff muscles, improves circulation and, through the action of the deep-seated muscles associated with the breathing, stimulates the internal systems of the body.

Just a word of caution – intriguing as the imagery of the Serpent Goddess and the lotus centres of energy along the axis of the spine may be, it comes from an age and a culture far distant from the Western developed world, where it is only a concept of the imagination.

Anyone who sits still to practise Pranayama or meditation will experience, at times, a rebalance of mechanical forces and a release of energy. These subjective personal experiences only become confused and self-important if associated with unreal objects of fantasy and ambition. Images which may be valid symbols for integration in their time and place can be doors to psychotic states for those born in different ages, cultures and continents.

> When thy mind leaves behind its dark forest of delusion, thou shalt go beyond the scriptures of times past and still to come. (*Bhagavad Gita*, 2, 52.)

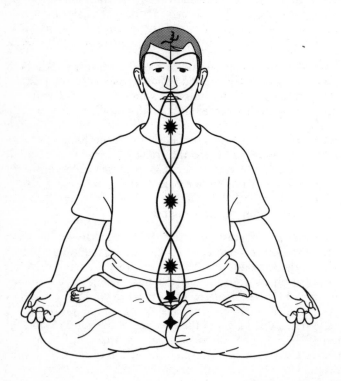

The chakras are named:

1 Mooladhara – base of sacrum
2 Svadhishthana – genitals
3 Manipura – navel
4 Anahata – heart
5 Visudaha – throat
6 Ajnapura – between eyebrows
7 Sahasvara – crown of head.

With the invasion of India by the colonial powers her religious practices and philosophies eventually became known further afield. The Scriptures, originally written in Sanskrit and therefore read only by the priestly caste, the Brahmins, were translated and became available for study more widely. The latter half of the nineteenth century saw an increase in Eastern religion and philosophy, including Yoga, in the West. Indian teachers began to travel to the West, notably Vivekananda (1863–1902). He was a disciple of the great Hindu saint Ramakrishna (1836–86). There has been a continuing interest in Yoga shown this century, particularly during the late 1960s and early 1970s. Many gurus travelled to the West in search of pupils, some finding fame and fortune and there was a steady traffic from West to East of people searching for a teacher.

The way that Yoga is handed down from guru to disciple has meant that a wide spectrum of teaching is inevitable, and at the present time there are schools of Yoga of every imaginable kind, from exercise classes to extreme, dangerous cults. It is in the esoteric writings that the guidance of a Teacher is said to be essential for the very involved secret procedures they advocate. In the *Yoga Sutras* the need for a guru is not mentioned. Vivekananda in his book *Raja Yoga* wrote 'Anything secret or mysterious in the systems of Yoga should be rejected ... mystery-mongering weakens the human brain. It has well nigh destroyed Yoga, one of the grandest sciences.'

One tradition is that you will find a teacher when you are truly in need of one. In today's world of mass communication it seems to be more a case of sorting your way through the volume of people begging to instruct you. That said, when you really need someone, there are real teachers to be found. They, however, are a gift and can be neither sought nor bought.

02

teach yourself through practice

In this chapter you will learn:
- the preliminary requirements for practice
- common sense rules for Yoga postures
- basic rules for practice.

Yoga can only be understood through practice. You have to try it for yourself in order to learn what it is really about. You cannot look at the pictures of the Asanas or read about meditation and know what they are. It is only by discovering them for yourself that you will have a chance of finding their purpose.

Practice demands commitment. It requires time and attention if you are going to do Yoga regularly, so it is not something to be started casually.

In the *Yoga Sutras* Patanjali gives three preliminary requirements for anyone starting Yoga. These are: Tapas (Austerity), Svadhyaya (Study) and Isvara-Pranidhana (Surrender to God).

Tapas

Tapas translated from the Sanskrit as 'Austerity' seems, at first, a rather unattractive idea for most of us. If you are going to start Yoga, say the *Sutras*, you have to be prepared to have some order in your life. The word Tapas, which is also one of Patanjali's five personal disciplines (Niyamas) of the second of the eight steps, contains the idea of heat, a burning away of the unnecessary things in our lives so that we live more simply. Regular Yoga practice will tend to make you lead a more disciplined life, not just in the time put aside for practice itself, but in the effect the practice will have on your day-to-day existence. The practice of Asanas alone can change your attitude to your body as you become aware of the effects of food, alcohol and smoking, and the practice of relaxation Pranayama and Meditation reduces our need for endless distractions and we become more discriminating in what we listen to on the radio or how often we watch television. Tapas does not mean extreme fasting, beds of nails or depriving yourself of sleep; as the *Bhagavad Gita* explains 'Yoga is a harmony. Not for him who eats too much, or for him who eats too little; not for him who sleeps too little or for him who sleeps too much.' Tapas should lead to a balanced life and not to disorder.

Svadhyaya

Svadhyaya can be interpreted as the study of sacred texts, the acquiring of self-knowledge, and also the repetition of the name of God as a form of meditation (Japa). Repetition must be accompanied by reflection on the meaning of the sacred word.

Isvara Pranidhana

Isvara Pranidhana means making God the motive for our actions. A belief in God is part of classical Yoga, which is one of the philosophical systems of Hinduism. The teaching of the Buddha fell outside Hinduism because his path to Nirvana did not entail any such belief, as well as rejecting the caste system and the authority of the *Vedas*. In Yoga the fruits of our actions should not be for ourselves but for the service of God. Of course Asanas, Pranayama and Meditation can be practised by anybody for any motive, but to be truely Yoga in the strict sense, a belief in God is necessary, as Yoga is in essence a religious path. The *Bhagavad Gita* says that we should offer God the practice of Yoga, sacred studies, knowledge and the out-flowing and in-flowing breath.

When you start to practise Yoga it does not matter if you are young or old, an athlete or disabled. The moment that you decide to begin contains in it all that you need. Within each of us at that moment is the blueprint, or map, of the path we can take, a different path for each person. The preliminaries of Yoga practice are a means of finding our place on that map and clearing away through discipline, study and renunciation some of the rubbish that obscures the way forward. Finding our place on the map is important because most people have no idea where they are when they start, very often imagining themselves to be steadier and in a better state of awareness than in fact they are. For example, on a physical level, you may find that the flexibility that you had imagined to be an advantage in the postures turns out to be a disadvantage if you lack strength and stability. Yoga practice may bring humility but on the other hand, false humility that ignores or refuses to accept our strengths and sensitivities must also fall away. Hence the need for the self-knowledge of Svadhyaya.

Asanas

The body is the index, the outward sign, the clue as to where to begin. 'Sit still ...', says the *Bhagavad Gita* 'with head and neck erect' and only then 'fix your heart on the One Supreme'.

Each body is different in proportion, in physical type, in how it adapts to stress, and the gifts with which it was born; the way that we should practise will, to a certain extent, be different for each one of us.

At the moment health crazes and fitness crazes abound, trainers and therapists help us pursue often illusory goals of physical and psychological excellence, many of them taking us further and further away from where we should truly stand. When we practise Asanas we have to dismiss from our minds the fashionable concepts of fitness. Yoga, as we have seen, is extremely old and has very little in common with modern aerobic exercise and weight training. Some modern Yoga teachers, anxious to justify their subject, distort the teaching by adapting it to present day thinking. This is a pity because Yoga has stood the test of time, Yogis being renowned for their superb health and longevity, while some of the excessive training methods of modern athletes are being shown to be so stressful that they can damage the body and cause illness.

Yoga practice is about economy of energy; it has nothing to do with 'working out'. You shouldn't feel tired after Yoga, nor should you experience a 'high' followed by exhaustion a few hours later. Rather practice should increase your energy and potential for life from day to day.

Yoga Asanas have evolved over thousands of years as a way of 'undoing' the stiffness and tensions of the body, of strengthening its weaknesses and restoring equilibrium. This is done mainly through stretching and readjusting the balance of the spine, the body's structural and neurological core. Although some of the more complicated postures may look bizarre to the uninitiated, Asanas are not about struggling to impose a seemingly impossible contortion on the body, but are a way of restoring it through the use of breathing, stability and the release of the spine.

Common sense rules of Asana practice

Before we start to practise there are some basic rules that we should know – natural rules of common sense. All the exercises are perfectly safe if you do them without aggression and follow the instructions carefully bearing these basic rules in mind. If you are in any doubt, you should consult a qualified medical practioner before attempting them.

The spine

The spinal column is the basic support of the body and within its protective channel run the main nerves to and from the brain. All your bodily functions as well as movement depend on these nerves.

A baby in its mother's womb lies curled up so that at birth the spine is in one long outward curve. As a child learns to lift its head and crawl and walk, the inward curves of the neck and waist develop so that by the time she or he is an adult the spine is balanced in four opposing curves.

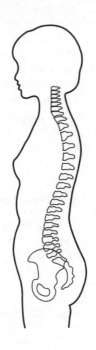

The lowest curve of the spine is the composite bone of the sacrum formed of five fixed vertebrae fused together with the rudimentary 'tail' of the coccyx beneath it. The sacrum forms the back of the pelvis or hip girdle as it fits between the two ilia bones, which flare out and curve round to meet at the pubic symphasis at the front. The ischias bones (or sitting bones), which we can feel under our buttocks when we sit are the lowest part of the pelvis. These are the 'roots' in all the sitting poses.

The pelvis and the sacrum are designed for strength, but above the sacrum the spine is made up of movable vertebrae with discs of cartilage between them to act as shock absorbers and make the spine elastic. The vertebrae are all slightly different from each other: the five lumbar vertebrae just above the sacrum are very thick and strong – they have a lot of weight to carry and fit above one another in a way that only allows a little twisting or backwards movement. The twelve thoracic vertebrae, which carry the ribs, are lighter and more mobile; the ribcage needs to be elastic as well as protective as it contains the lungs and heart. The cervical vertebrae of the neck are the lightest of all with a big range of movement. At the back and sides of the vertebrae there are bony spines or processes protecting the spinal cord, which runs from the brain and is the main pathway of the nervous system.

Your spine needs to be both strong and flexible. If you have perfect posture the weight of your head balances effortlessly at the top of your neck; as you move the whole spinal column adjusts and readjusts adapting to the force of gravity easily, freely, gracefully so that movement entails a minimum of effort and there is no feeling of tension. Should you want to stand or sit completely still to meditate or practise Pranayama, the head ribcage and pelvis should balance one above the other with no strain on the muscles of the back or shoulders. It is in order to maintain, or more likely regain, this happy state of perfect postural balance and bodily mechanical efficiency that you need to practise Yoga Asanas, which should always allow the natural curves of the spine space to elongate and readjust.

The bones of the skeleton are bound together by ligaments and enveloped by layers of muscles that continually stretch and contract as you move. Without you being aware of it your natural sense of balance, and proprioceptive sense, will ensure that your muscles continually tighten and release to hold you upright against the force of gravity that pulls us towards the centre of the earth. Unfortunately, for many of us, the repeated restricted movements of modern daily life and habitual mannerisms tend to distort our posture. Muscles that should be contracting and releasing have to tighten continually to hold a misaligned part of the body in place and the symmetry of the spinal curves become distorted.

This question of good postural balance should be important for us all, many people can get away with slumping about and not caring too much how they stand and sit, but if you want to sit still and practise Pranayama or meditation, and if you are suffering from ill-health or backache, then how your spine moves becomes vitally important. To sit still, even when we sit well, is a strain on the body for bodies are made to move and move we must if we are to stay healthy and our digestive system, circulation and other bodily functions are to work properly.

Asanas move the body in many different directions and this, together with breathing, stimulates not only the muscles and joints but the circulation, digestion, nervous and endocrine systems, which govern our health and vitality.

Breath

Asanas are not just an exercise of the muscles equalizing their tone and efficiency. Asanas are done with the exhalation of the breath, the movement is always a release away from the centre of the body to the periphery, an elongation and an outward release. This is true even in positions where the body appears to curl up such as Crane Pose (page 68), or Tortoise Pose (page 57).

The diaphragm, which contracts and relaxes as we breathe, lies inside the trunk across the bottom of the ribcage; at the back its fibres extend far down the front of the lumbar spine (waist) where they meet the ilio psoas muscles, which also run along the front of the spine going down right through the back of the pelvis into the tops of the femurs (upper leg bones).

These inner spinal muscles are important for postural alignment as they integrate the legs with the spine and affect the curve of the waist and the tilt of the pelvis. As you breathe out these inner spinal muscles should release with the diaphragm allowing the curve at the back of the waist to lengthen. The abdominal muscles, which contract on exhalation, balance this release at the back of the waist so that the lumbar spine lengthens and the pelvis drops down away from the waist if you are standing or sitting. There is therefore a moment when the spine lengthens naturally with the exhalation that allows you do Asanas without effort. The inhalation should always be quiet as we should never 'take' a breath but receive it gently.

Gravity

The *Yoga Sutras* say that Asana should be 'stable and relaxed' and that this may be achieved by 'relaxation of effort and concentration on the infinite'. The root of the Sanskrit word

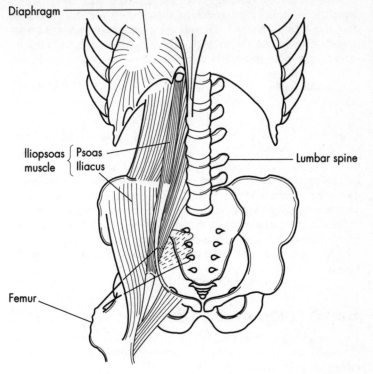

Diaphragm

Iliopsoas muscle { Psoas
Iliacus

Lumbar spine

Femur

which is translated as 'infinite' is 'Ananta'. In Hindu mythology Ananta is the serpent with a thousand heads whose power holds the universe in its place; the serpent who forms the resting place of the God, Vishnu. Patanjali, writer of the *Yoga Sutras*, was reputed to have been one of the incarnations of Ananta. The word is also translated as fixity. This concept of being in contact with the power that holds the earth so that the body is secure to relax is vital to understanding the practice of Yoga poses, for the downward pull of gravity is counteracted by the impulse of all living things to expand and grow upwards. Each Yoga Asana has to be done in accordance with this double action of stability and freedom.

Asanas use the force of gravity to stabilize the base of the pose so the spinal column can elongate with the exhalation of the breath; this is a natural, spontaneous release of tension that has nothing to do with performance, aggression or control but is a rediscovery of the joy of movement and physical freedom.

When you stand erect, aligned and balanced with the force of gravity the head, chest and hips should be over each other so that the four curves of the spine balance each other without distortion. The line of gravity, which can be demonstrated by dropping a plumbline, should pass through the centre of the head behind the ears, through the tops of the shoulders, hip joints, the knees and the ankles. When you stand straight the centre of gravity is inside the hip girdle at the level of the top of the sacrum.

Yoga Asanas have to be done with these three things in mind. Stability is achieved through the force of gravity so that there is no tension and the minimum effort is expended. The spine must lengthen, even in the most complicated poses so that every movement can release and readjust any distortions. This release and lengthening of the spine comes through using the breath, there being a movement at the end of the exhalation when the body can stretch spontaneously, like the movement of a wave which, if taken at the right moment, takes a surfer far up the beach.

Basic rules in practice

Each pose has its roots which go down into the earth and hold us steady and secure so that we can release and stretch without effort or tension.

When we are standing these roots are our heels. In inverted poses such as headstand, shoulderstand or handstand they are the elbows or the hands. In sitting positions the roots are the sitting bones (ischias bones). With stability at the base of the pose the spine can lengthen as you breathe, releasing the pelvis away from the the back of the waist and the head away from the neck. This means that the spine is not compressed and distorted as you do the poses but frees itself from any habitual imbalances as it moves. The spine releases and lengthens in all the Asanas, even the seemingly complicated ones. In backbends, for example, the spine lengthens in order to bend, it does not just hinge in the back of the waist and even in twisting movements the spine must lengthen in order to turn.

In the beginning you have to start with simple poses where the experience of being stable and grounded at the base of the pose can be felt easily. The instructions for these poses are marked with one asterisk (*). When you have become stable and can stretch with the movement of the breath you can begin to understand the purpose of the more complicated postures, which are a further means of helping you 'undo' tensions as you stretch and balance with the breath. These poses are marked with two asterisks (**). Until you feel the need to go further in your practice **keep it simple**. It is possible to do any of the poses by pushing into them and compressing the curves of the spine as it bends; this can enable you to do the pose but eventually your body becomes tired and stressed and this road comes to an end. Yogis, unlike dancers and gymnasts, should be still practising and improving in their 80s and 90s.

Doing difficult poses is not a sign of being 'advanced', and if you find something hard you could be trying it too soon. Body types vary so much that there may be some poses that will never be appropriate for you, though the boundaries of possibility will almost certainly not be where you imagined them to be before you started Yoga. The more difficult poses marked with three asterisks (***) will not be suitable for everyone and are best learned with the help of a teacher.

According to Yoga philosophy the whole of creation is subject to the three influences of Rajas (activity), Tamas (inertia) and Sattva (clarity), known collectively as the Gunas. It is only when these are in balance that liberation is possible. As you practise Yoga you come to understand the fluctuations of these tendencies in your body and in your breathing as well as in other aspects of everyday existence.

When you stop trying to 'do' the pose, you have a chance of finding true stillness and stability in the pull of gravity, which gives you the chance to follow the rise and fall of the current of the breath as you extend into the pose. This is a discovery of inner strength and energy which is completely different from that which we normally use. As Yoga postures are the result of this 'letting go' through using the breath, and not the result of effort and struggle, normal physical limits do not apply. Sometimes we hear of Yogis who can stop their heart beat, raise their body temperature in freezing conditions or allow themselves to be buried in the ground. These kind of results and curiosities are, however, never the aim of serious practice, although sometimes Yogis' techniques are used to bring about these supranormal states deliberately. The extreme results of this type of exploitation bring Yoga into disrepute, just as the misuse of drugs or surgery can bring modern medicine into disrepute.

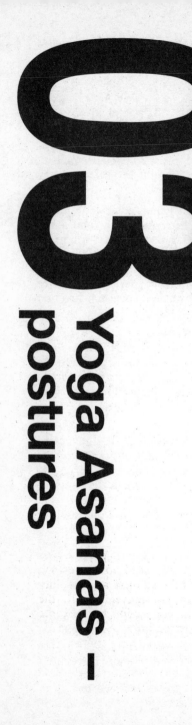

03

Yoga Asanas – postures

In this chapter you will learn:
- the Yoga Asanas
- the postures in detail
- the Sun Salute sequence
- relaxation techniques.

Standing straight (Tadasana)*

Standing straight is the easiest way to experience the basic principles of Yoga Asanas. This is why it is the first Asana that you will learn and the first to be practised. To be able to stand straight and erect, steady and relaxed is the aim of all Yoga Asana practice. This is the key to sitting to meditate.

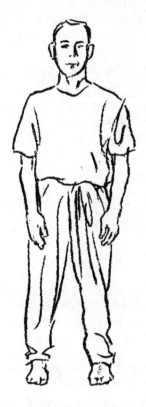

Each Asana has a Sanskrit name. Asana means posture and Tada means mountain and this is the key as to how to do the pose. Tada the mountain symbolizes the stillness and stability which is the beginning and end of all movement. In the macrocosm Tada symbolizes also the connection between the earth below and the heavens above, in the microcosm the spine along which the energy centres of the subtle body are aligned, the source of our health and energy. All the other Asanas are but a means of balancing and adjusting the physical structure so that Tadasana can be performed perfectly. In this pose as in sitting meditative poses it is not just the physical body that is still and relaxed, there is also an inner balance of alertness and tranquillity, of sensitivity and strength that brings clarity.

1 Stand with your feet slightly apart and parallel.
2 Feel your weight on your heels.
3 Keep your knees straight.
4 As you exhale feel your weight being pulled down towards the floor through your heels while from the waist you grow upwards towards the sky.
5 Keep your shoulders and arms relaxed.
6 Your feet must be completely stable and the backs of your knees should stretch without consciously tightening the thigh muscles. (See notes on feet in Chapter 7, Therapeutic uses of Yoga Asanas and Pranayama.)

Standing poses

The easiest and safest way to let your spine release with the exhalation is from a standing position. As you walk you should be able to move easily and spontaneously with strong feet and legs, relaxed shoulders and arms, and with your spine adjusting and readjusting to the pull of gravity. Unfortunately many of us have lost this ability, as most daily tasks in modern life tend to make us tense and tight in the shoulders and out of touch with our contact with the earth through our feet.

In all these poses be aware of your heels (or heel) being firmly anchored down on the ground so that from the secure base you can exhale and lengthen into the pose. Take time and wait for the moment in the exhalation when there is a natural impulse for your body to release and stretch.

You can stay in the poses as long as you can release tension and lengthen with each exhalation. If you find yourself contracting and becoming rigid to 'hold onto' a pose you have kept it for too long. This rule applies to all Yoga Asanas.

Tree pose (Vrksasana) *

A tree has its roots deep in the earth while the trunk and branches reach upwards. Standing on one leg in this pose, feel that you are drawn onto the straight plumbline of gravity so the foot and hips become more and more rooted down and the spine lengthens upwards.

It is more important to be properly aligned in this position than it is to stand unsupported, so at the beginning stand near a wall and use it to keep your balance.

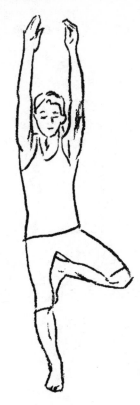

1 Start standing straight in mountain pose to feel the correct balance.
2 Keep your weight on the heel of the standing foot and exhale as you fold the other leg letting the thigh rotate outwards, place the heel of the raised foot as high on the inside of the standing leg as you can.
3 Keep your neck and shoulders relaxed so that your head finds its natural balance, and then with another out breath stretch your arms upwards above your head.
4 Repeat the pose on the other side.

The understanding of stability and balance learned through the practice of this pose is important when it comes to learning headstand.

Tree pose in lotus (Ardha Padma Padottanasana) **

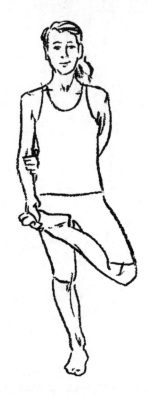

Eagle pose (Garudasana) **

This is another balancing pose and, like the other bird pose (Crane Pose, page 68) there is a feeling of being pulled towards the centre as the exhalation contracts the abdomen and the spine lengthens.

1 Stand straight, then standing on the right leg with an exhalation swing the left leg across the front of the right thigh and tuck the foot behind your lower right leg as in the picture. To do this your right leg will have to bend a

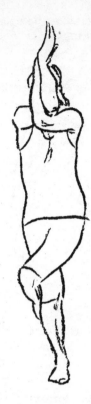

little. Your weight stays on your heel and the back of the waist stays long.

2 Exhale again and cross your right elbow over your left one and then wrap your lower arms round each other so that the palms are facing.

3 Stay in the pose for a few breaths and then repeat on the other side. Beginners should practise the arm movement only to start with (see page 125, Chapter 7).

Warrior pose (Virabhadrasana) *

This pose extends from the original standing position into another one-legged balance. As your weight shifts from one leg to the other your spine stays long, and there is a stretch from the back heel to the fingertips. This evolving, lengthening balance brings a feeling of great stability and growing strength, controlled and powerful, but not aggressive.

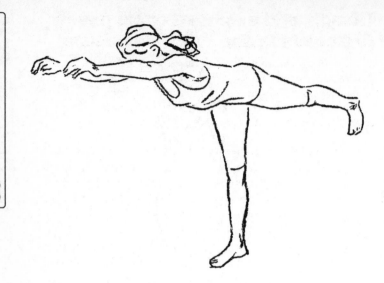

1 Stand straight.
2 Exhale and step one foot a walking pace forwards, keeping your weight on your back foot.
3 Raise your arms over your head without tightening your shoulders.
4 Exhale and lengthen forwards and upwards from the hips towards your fingertips letting your weight come onto your front foot as your back leg comes off the ground, your back knee stays straight as your back leg stretches away from your trunk as it lifts up.
5 Continue to lengthen with each exhalation as your back leg comes further up and your arms stretch forwards. With practice your back leg, arms and hands will be horizontal.
6 Stay for a few breaths and then with an exhalation let your back leg drop so the foot resumes its original place, one step behind the other one. The straight line from the back heel to the hands stays constant throughout.
7 Repeat the pose on the other side.

Triangle and extended angle poses (Trikonasana and Parsvakonasana) *

In these poses the spine twists and extends sideways. The back heel remains firmly on the floor and the back leg stays straight. With the hips stabilized by the anchor of the back foot the spine lengthens towards your head. Your shoulders should stay relaxed so that your arms can extend freely.

1 Take a long step forwards from the standing straight pose. Keep your feet pointing forwards and your weight on the back heel. The distance between the feet depends on how tall you are and the length of your legs. If the distance is too short you will not have a long enough base for the pose to be secure. If, however, the distance is too long then you will not be able to keep your weight anchored down on your back heel as you go into the position.

2 Exhale and turn towards your back leg extending your arms to the side.

3 With another out breath stretch out to the side and, keeping your weight on your back heel, go down so

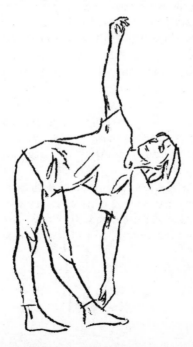

that your lower arm rests behind your leg. Be careful that you don't bend forwards; your head should be in line with your front foot.

4 Stay for a few breaths and then come up with an exhalation. Your back heel stays anchored down throughout.

5 Repeat on the other side.

When this pose is done with both legs straight so that they make a triangle with the floor this pose is called Trikonasana or triangle pose. You can also practise it allowing the front knee to bend while keeping your weight on the back heel. You will be able to go a bit further in this position but it is more difficult to stay grounded on the back heel, which is essential for the release along the spine. When the front knee is bent the pose is called extended angle pose (Parsvakonasana).

Triangle twist and extended angle twist (Parivrtta Trikonasana and Parivrtta Pasvakonasana)*

In these poses that rotate the spine it is difficult to stay grounded on the back heel so go slowly and practise the straight poses first.

Start as in the simple poses but at step 2 turn towards the front foot so that your trunk twists round across the line of the pelvis. Keep your back heel firmly down as you exhale.

Standing forward bend (Uttanasana) *

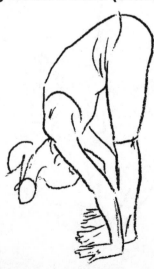

1 Stand straight.

2 Exhale and bend forwards keeping your knees straight. If your hands don't reach the floor, stretch forwards and let them rest on a table instead. Your spine needs space to lengthen forwards and the back of your legs will need some time to stretch. Go slowly, you have everything to gain by doing this pose with support for some months. It is more important to lengthen than it is to touch the floor.

3 Stay in the pose for several breaths. Your heels should stay down and your hips should be vertically over your feet. Keep your shoulders relaxed.

4 Come up with an exhalation keeping your weight on your heels.

Wide astride pose (Prasarita Padottanasana) *

This pose is similar to the standing forward bend except that the feet are wide apart, they remain parallel with the weight on the outside of the heels. It is easier to touch the ground with the legs wide, but if you have a problem then stretch forwards to a support as in the previous pose.

Triangle forward bend (Parsvottanasana) *

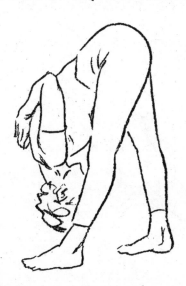

This is another forward bend but here your hands are folded up behind your back with the palms together and the fingers pointing upwards towards your neck in the prayer position. With your hands like this you can feel what is happening to your upper back as you bend forwards. It should be lengthening and not stooping forwards and shortening.

Start this forward bend by taking one foot a good step forwards while keeping your weight on your back heel. This will ensure that you feel secure as you bend forwards with your hands behind your back. Keep both legs straight and lengthen forwards with each exhalation as in the previous forward bends.

When you have practised Yoga for some time and can bend forwards easily keeping your weight firmly planted on your heels you can practise the standing forward bend and the wide astride pose with the hands folded up the back. In this position, this gives a good release to the shoulders and upper back.

Dog pose 1 (Svanasana) *

This is the stretch that a dog makes when it gets up after being asleep. As in the standing poses the heels go down and the knees straighten to anchor the hips and let the spine extend. This is a good release for the neck and shoulders before practising the inverted poses.

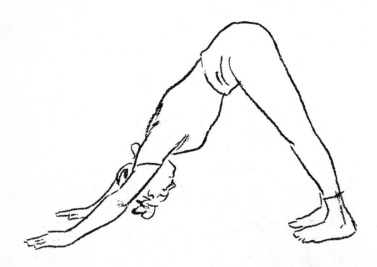

1 Kneel on all fours with your hands under your shoulders and your knees under your hips.
2 Tuck your toes under your heels, extending the soles of your feet. Spread out your fingers so that there is a good contact between your palms and the floor.
3 With an exhalation straighten your legs and extend your hips up and back away from your hands.
4 Do not tighten your shoulders, just let your heels go further down to the ground. With each exhalation let your back grow longer while your shoulders relax.

5 Stay for a few breaths and then come back to the all fours position and then without moving your hands sit back on your heels letting your trunk fold forwards. This folded pose is called child pose (Pindasana) and can be used for relaxation. If this is uncomfortable because your knees or feet are stiff, see pages 121 and 122 in Chapter 7.

Dog pose 2 **

The second part of the dog's stretch is a backbending movement. When you have mastered the first dog pose read the instructions for backbends on page 64 before trying this more difficult pose.

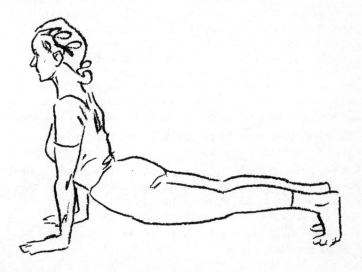

5 From step 4 of dog pose 1, exhale and, keeping your arms and legs straight, slowly drop your hips down towards the floor so that your spine bends backwards and your shoulders move forwards and up until they are over your wrists.

6 Your knees must stay straight so that your back thigh muscles pull the back of the pelvis downwards and the crease of the buttocks becomes strong. There should be no feeling of pinching at the back of the waist.

7 Your weight should be on your wrists and feet. Your knees, which are straight, stay above the ground. Keep your chin in to lengthen the back of the neck.

This is not a pose for beginners, who should practise the locust pose on page 64 first so that they understand how to lengthen the upper back when the spine extends in a backbend.

Inverted poses

The inverted poses give a feeling of balance and energy. When you do them properly they are wonderful positions in which to correct postural inbalances, to work injured knees or arthritic hips, and to restore yourself at the end of a hard day. Done badly, before you have understood, through practice, the basic principles of Yoga Asanas, they can cause problems as they are more difficult than the standing poses. When you go into these poses there can be a tendency to tighten the shoulders and push as you lift up into headstand or shoulderstand; this compresses the neck, where the vertebrae are small and mobile and the base of the pose becomes unstable. It is therefore vital that you prepare to go into these poses carefully making sure that you are straight before you go up, and allowing gravity to pull your elbows down into the ground so that the shoulders can release.

The whole pose must be rooted down through the elbows so that the spine is free to lengthen and balance as you breathe.

Caution: If you suffer from high blood pressure, glaucoma, detached retina, heart or circulatory problems, or any other condition that might make going upside down a problem, consult a doctor before attempting these poses.

For these poses you need a firm soft base, so use a folded blanket or towel.

Headstand (Sirsasana) **

The concentration of balance, breath and the reversal of the pull of gravity make headstand an extremely strong pose. It is sometimes known as the 'King' of the Asanas. When you practise it should always be followed by the more relaxing shoulderstand or 'Mother' of the Asanas.

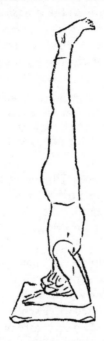

1 Kneel down and put your elbows on the blanket, shoulder width apart.
2 Link your fingers together and turn your wrists inwards towards your thumbs. The little fingers will slightly separate and the palms turn down.

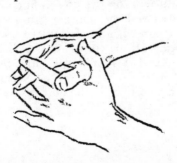

3 Take time to relax your shoulders, letting your elbows drop down to the ground. Your little fingers and wrists should stretch away from your elbows making a firm triangular base. This base must stay still and down throughout.

4 Drop your head so that the centre of the crown rests on the floor in the centre of the triangle formed by the elbows and wrists.

5 Straighten your legs. Your elbows stay down and your hips should be in line with your head so that the spine stretches up vertically.

This is the point where you can adjust your position safely. If you are practising by yourself you can use a mirror so that you can look between your legs and check that your head, neck and hips are symmetrical. The mirror must reach down to the floor and be vertical.

6 Exhale, and keeping your elbows down, bend your knees and take your feet off the floor. Do not swing your hips backwards but let the whole spine from the skull to the hips lengthen upwards. Keep your neck long.

7 Exhale again and slowly let your legs straighten upwards until you are vertical.

Concentrate on keeping your elbows down so that the base of the pose stays secure. Each time you breathe out, feel your body finding its centre of gravity so that eventually you can balance without effort.

8 To come down, exhale and bend your knees and come down as you went up. Finish by kneeling forwards on the floor with your head dropped down so that your neck relaxes. (Child pose, page 51.)

Beginners: The best way to do this pose is in the centre of the room. If you are near a wall the tendency is to keep touching it with your feet for support when you feel insecure so that you get into the habit of being off the correct vertical line of balance. Once you have acquired this habit it is difficult to learn to balance properly. If you need support at the beginning, practise headstand in a corner so that the support is evenly placed on both sides of you.

You can stay in headstand for some minutes as long as the base of the pose remains stable and your body is lengthening and adjusting to the pull of gravity each time you exhale. If the pose feels 'locked' and stiff, or if the back of your waist or neck are collapsing, come down immediately.

Shoulderstand (Sarvangasana) *

Shoulderstand is learned before headstand and can be practised on its own. This is a quiet relaxing pose once you have learned to go into it without compressing your neck or tightening your shoulders.

Caution: People with problems in the neck can try the modified position described on page 120 in Chapter 7.

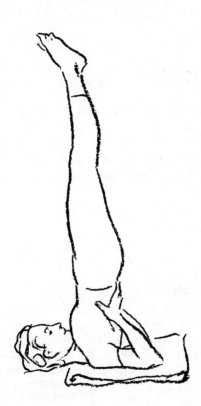

As with headstand, make sure you are straight before you go into the pose; any adjustment has to be done at the beginning when you are lying on the floor. Once you are up in the position do not move your head; if you think you are crooked come down and start again.

1 Lie flat on your back with your knees bent. The folded blanket should be under your shoulders and your elbows. Be sure that your head is straight. Your arms should be by your side with your palms down. Stay in this position for several breaths letting your arms release towards your feet.

2 Exhale and roll your hips and spine up off the floor taking your feet over your head. Your arms stay on the floor behind you. Beginners should have a chair behind them so that their feet can rest on that instead of going all the way down to the floor.

Caution: When you roll your feet over your head do not push with your arms and shoulders or tense your neck.

3 Keeping your elbows down on the ground, put your hands on your back so that your back ribs are supported by your palms and wrists. Make sure that your head and trunk are straight. This position is the plough pose. Your legs should be straight and your spine long.

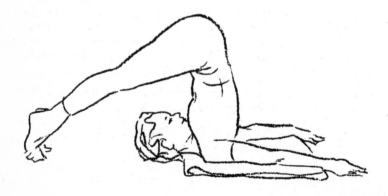

4 Exhale and take your legs up so that your whole body from your shoulders to your feet is in a straight vertical line. Your weight should be on your elbows which stay down on the floor.

5 To come down take the feet back to plough pose, put your hands on the floor with the palms down and, keeping your shoulders relaxed, roll slowly down without lifting your head from the floor. Go slowly and take several breaths to do this so that your spine uncurls along the floor. To begin with bend your knees as you do this. Later you can do it with straight legs.

Beginners: At first you may find it difficult to lift up so that you are in a straight vertical shoulderstand. Keeping your weight on your elbows come up as far as you can and after a few breaths take your feet back onto the chair behind your head and roll gently down so that you are lying flat on the floor. Gradually as your body and particularly your upper back loosens up you will be able to go up higher. Your elbows must stay on the floor all the time and there should be no feeling of pressure in the face or neck.

Once you are able to do the full vertical pose you can stay in the position for some minutes. This should be a calming, resting pose that relieves stiffness round the shoulders, neck and upper spine. It is a good recuperation pose at the end of a hard day.

Variations
When you are upside down, the hips and legs bear no weight. Once the pose is secure, you can move completely differently as you are unrestricted by the normal pull of gravity. These further inverted poses are a natural evolution of the feeling of release and strength that a good headstand or shoulderstand brings. They should be practised with that in mind and never as an end in themselves.

To do these poses the 'roots' of the basic position must be stable and the spine must be free to elongate.

Single leg headstand (Ekapada Sirsasana) ***

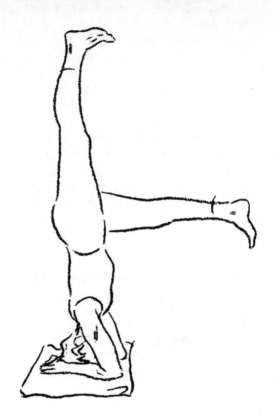

Single leg shoulderstand (Ekapada Sarvangasana) **

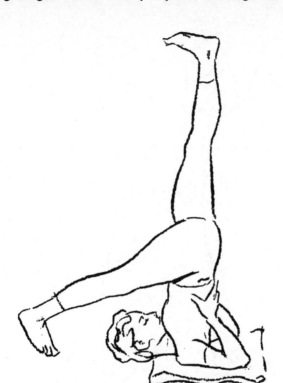

Maintenance of the basic position is the key to these poses, so the leg that remains uppermost continues to elongate upwards along the line of balance allowing the descending leg to act as a counterweight.

Lotus in headstand (Urdhva Padmasana in Sirsasana) ***

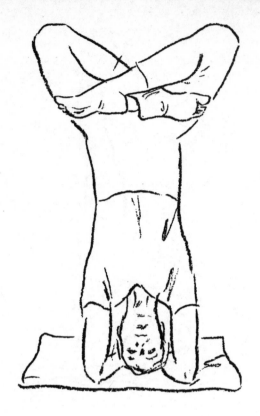

Lotus in shoulderstand (Urdhva Padmasana in Sarvangasana) ***

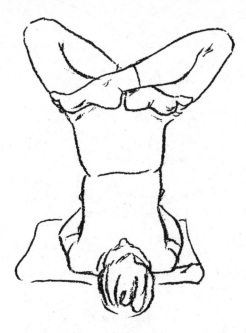

In these poses the knees should be close to one another so that the pelvis lifts and extends away from the waist. The fish pose (page 60) must be learned first before these poses are attempted.

In shoulderstand you can use your hands to pull your legs into lotus pose. In headstand you need to be able to do lotus without using your hands; this will require a certain degree of flexibility and some practice. In these variations, as in the others the head and neck stay in the original position, the elbows stay down and the spine and legs stretch away from the trunk.

Plough pose with the knees to the ears (Karnapidasana) **

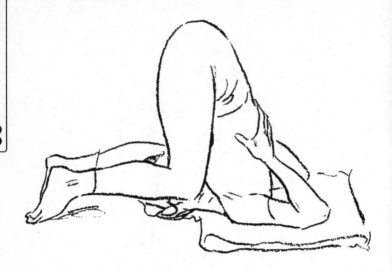

This variation of plough pose gives a big stretch to the upper back and neck; it is one of the positions where body proportions play a big role. If you have a long spine and short legs it will be more difficult to touch your knees to the floor; remember the Asana is not there to be achieved but should be a help to the body. Go as far as feels good and don't push; your elbows (as always) stay down.

Supine poses

If you are tired at the end of the day you can start your practice with these supine poses, otherwise practise them after the inverted poses as you will get a better movement when your weight has been off your legs for a bit.

Supine leg stretches (Supta Padangusthasana) *

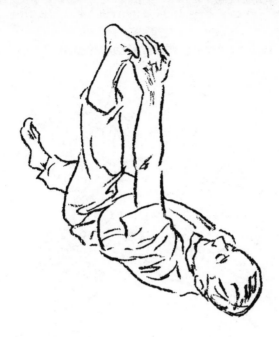

1 Lie on your back.
2 Bring one leg towards your chest with the knee bent, holding behind your thigh.
3 Exhale letting your abdomen go in and stretch the straight leg away from you. At the end of the breath bring the folded leg closer to your chest. This should be a release that comes with the breath, don't tighten your shoulders and pull.
4 Stay like this for several breaths, then straighten the folded leg and catch hold of the foot. (If you have tight hamstrings and find this difficult, loop a belt round your foot and hold that.)
5 As you exhale, there should be a moment at the end of the breath where, as the abdomen goes down, the lower leg stretches away and your raised leg comes towards your chest.

Variation: Letting the raised leg turn outwards in the hip, take it down gently towards the ground. Go slowly with small circular movements. Repeat these movements on the other side.

Supine twist (Jatara Parivartanasana) *

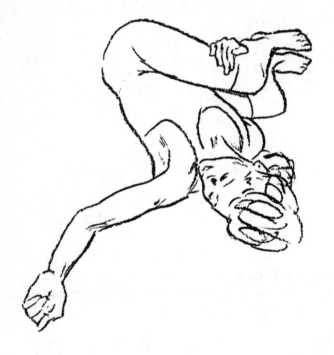

1 Lie on your back and hug your knees by holding behind your thighs. Keep all your back on the floor.
2 Keep your chin in and roll your head to the right letting your right arm drop to the floor.
3 Still hugging your legs to your chest exhale and roll your hips to the left. Your shoulders stay on the ground and your head stays to the right.
4 Then exhale and come back to the centre. Do the pose on the other side.

Variation: ** After you have twisted into the final position, stretch your legs straight; you should keep your thighs as close to your chest as possible. You can only do this if you have long hamstrings. If you find this difficult then wait and concentrate on doing the pose with the legs bent.

Sitting poses

When we sit, the 'sitting bones' (ischias tuberosities – the knobs beneath the pelvis under the buttocks) are the roots of the pose. In order for these to anchor firmly down when sitting on the floor you need to be flexible in the hip joints, which can be a problem for many Westerners accustomed to sitting on chairs. This is why the standing poses are more suitable for beginners than the sitting positions. If you find these poses difficult look in the therapy chapter on stiff hips on page 123.

There are a great many sitting poses in Yoga. The legs can be placed in a variety of ways in order to release the hips, but the basic movement is always the same. The pelvis starts straight so that the base of the pose is anchored down before the spine lengthens away from the hips.

Use a folded blanket to sit on.

Sitting forward bend (Paschimottanasana) *

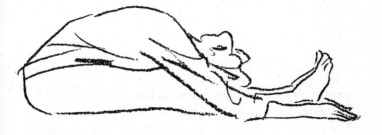

1 Sit on the floor with your legs straight out in front of you. To begin with you may have to tighten the front thigh muscles to straighten your knees, but in time, as you let the weight of your hips anchor down in order to bend forwards the legs will straighten without becoming tense.

2 Exhale and, keeping your shoulders relaxed, lengthen forwards to hold your feet with your hands. This movement must be from the spine so do not pull on your feet.

3 Exhale again and keeping your hips down, lengthen further forwards until the front of your trunk touches your legs. Don't try to touch your head to your legs, your spine should lengthen forwards not stoop over and shorten.

4 Stay for several breaths and then exhale and come up.

If you are flexible and have practised for some time you may find that you can relax quietly in this position and stay for up to ten minutes.

Beginners: If it is difficult to catch your feet, you can loop a belt round them and hold that instead.

Wide angle pose (Upavistha Konasana) *

This is a variation of the sitting forward bend.

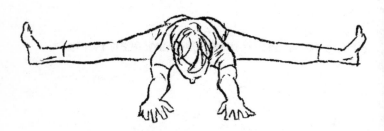

1 Sit with you legs wide apart and your knees facing the ceiling.

2 Do not let your legs roll inwards as you elongate forwards.

Thunderbolt pose (Vajrasana) *

This kneeling pose is suitable for Meditation or Pranayama practice.

1 Sit on your heels keeping your feet together and flat so that your pelvis is supported evenly by your heels. You

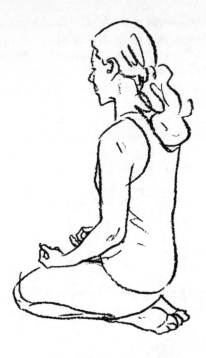

can put a rolled blanket under the tops of your feet if they are stiff. In time you will be able to dispense with this.

2 You should sit straight in this position with your head, shoulders and hips in a vertical line. Your shoulders are relaxed and your hands rest quietly on your thighs. When your feet and hips are flexible you can stay for a considerable period of time in this position.

Child pose (Pindasana) *

This folded forwards kneeling pose can be used as a relaxation position. It is also a useful recuperation, or counterpose, after headstand, dog pose or crane pose.

1 From thunderbolt pose exhale and keeping your sitting bones in contact with your heels extend forwards. At first your back may not lengthen enough to allow your head to touch the floor, so in this case put a cushion in front of you so that your head can rest easily (see page 127).

Hero pose (Virasana) *

In this kneeling pose your pelvis will tend to be tilted back a little. This makes it an unsuitable pose for Meditation or Pranayama as it will be difficult to maintain it for any length of time without collapsing your lower spine.

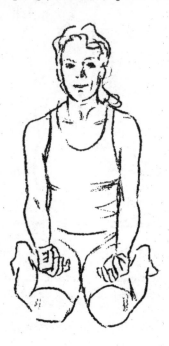

Sit on your heels as in thunderbolt pose and then, keeping your knees together, let your feet separate so that you are sitting on the floor between them with the soles of your feet facing the ceiling. Your sitting bones should be firmly down on the ground. This may be difficult at first, if so put a cushion between your feet and sit on that. As time goes by you will find that you are able to sit on the floor. If your feet are stiff and you get cramp put a rolled blanket or towel under them.

Caution: The front thighs need to stretch in this pose not the knees. If you feel any discomfort round the inside of the knee stop immediately and either use a higher cushion to sit on or wait a few more months before attempting this pose.

Bound angle pose (Baddha Konasana) *

This is the pose that appeared on the seals from the Indus valley 2000 BC.

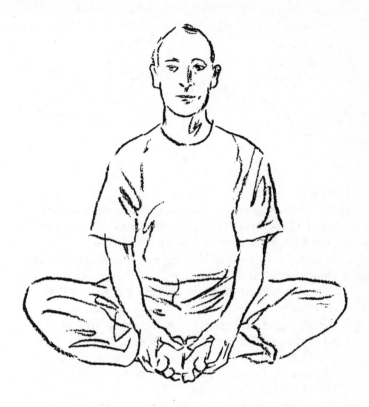

1 Sit with your legs apart as in wide angle pose.
2 Exhale and bend your knees and bring your feet as close in towards you as you can. Your thighs must turn out and your knees go down towards the floor.
3 Turn your feet so that the soles face the ceiling. If this is difficult at first practise by sitting with your back against a wall with a cushion under each thigh.
4 Let your thighs drop down towards the floor as you exhale letting the hips relax as you turn the feet out.
5 When your thighs drop right down to touch the floor you can lengthen forwards to touch your head to the floor.

Half bound angle pose (Janusirsasana) *

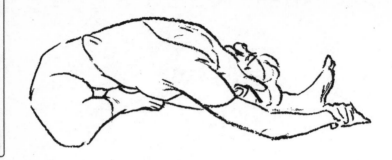

1 Sit with one leg straight in front of you and the other in bound angle pose. The base of this pose is not symmetrical so there is a tendency to sit crooked; both your sitting bones should be on the ground.

2 Keeping the hip of the bent leg well down exhale, and elongate that side of the spine first by extending that arm to hold the foot of the straight leg. This will give more stretch to one side of the back and pelvis.

3 Exhale again and stretch out the other arm as well allowing your spine to lengthen forwards. Either both hands should hold your extended foot or if you can lengthen far forwards you can catch your wrist beyond your foot as in the picture.

4 Come up and repeat on the other side. You may find that one side is stiffer than the other. If so, take more time in the earlier stages of the pose letting the hips release as you exhale.

Half hero pose (Triangmukhaikapada paschimottanasana) *

Sit with one leg straight out in front of you and the other folded back as in hero pose. This is another asymmetric pose, so follow the instructions for half bound angle pose.

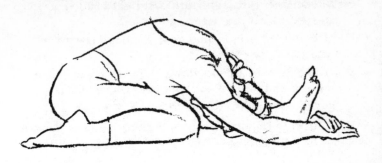

Sage's pose (Marichyasana) *

1 Sit on the ground with your left leg straight in front of you and your right leg bent up as if squatting. Your right heel should be close to your right buttock.

2 Extend forwards letting your right sitting bone come off the ground, let your left leg drop down as you exhale to reach forwards with your right arm. Keep your shoulders soft letting your right shoulder drop in front of your right knee.

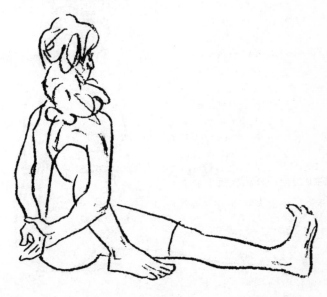

3 With another exhalation turn your right arm so that it entwines round your right leg.

4 Take you left arm behind your back and clasp your hands.

5 Drop both sitting bones down and exhaling lengthen upwards and turn to look over your left shoulder.

6 Stay for several breaths and repeat on the other side.

If this is hard to begin with stay in position 2 and continue to lengthen forwards.

Half lotus forward bend (Ardha Padma Paschimottanasana) **

1 Sit with one leg straight out in front of you and the other leg bent with the foot resting on the top of the opposite thigh as near to the groin as possible. (See the instructions for lotus on page 58.)

2 Keep your weight on the hip of the bent leg as you exhale and extend forwards on the bent leg side so that your hand catches the foot of the straight leg.

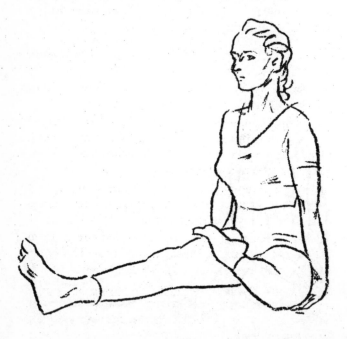

3 On another exhalation hold the foot with the other hand as well and continue to lengthen forwards with each ensuing outbreath. After several breaths come up and repeat the pose on the other side.

Tortoise pose (Kurmasana) **

There are two stages to this pose. First with the tortoise out of its shell and then asleep with its head and legs drawn in. You need supple shoulders as well as a good forward bending movement before you can get the benefit of this more difficult pose. It is not for beginners.

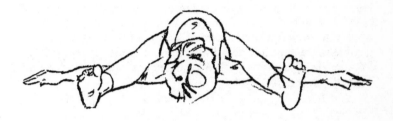

1 Sit with your knees bent up in front of you and your feet hip width apart.

2 Exhaling, stretch forwards letting your elbows drop to the ground between your legs.

3 When your shoulders are below your knees, turn one arm and then the other under your knees and extend them out along the ground with the palms facing down, at right angles to the body line.

4 As you exhale go further down letting the movement of your breath lengthen your back; first your forehead and then your chin will touch the ground.

5 Then, breathing out, turn your arms and stretch them backwards with the palms facing upwards. This is the tortoise with its legs and head out of its shell.

6 Extend your legs forwards and then bend your elbows and take your arms behind your back to hold your hands across your back ribs. (If you cannot hold your hands use a belt.)

7 Drop your hips down so that there is less pressure on your feet; draw your feet slightly towards you and cross your ankles one over the other.

8 Tuck your head into the little space between the ankles. This is sleeping tortoise (Supta Kurmasana).

Remember to practise this pose with the ankle crossed both ways.

You can stay for some time in this pose if it is comfortable and relaxing.

Lotus pose (Padmasana) **

This is the classic pose for sitting in meditation or for Pranayama. The hips are earthed to the floor, held by the weight of the feet on the thighs, so there is a secure base from which the spine can grow upwards and find its line of balance. If you are flexible in the hips and can do this pose it is the easiest position to hold for a long time, as it is completely steady, balanced and relaxed.

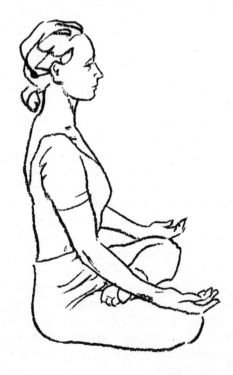

Caution: The movement in this position comes from the rotation of the thigh bone in the hip socket. The knee should bend normally and not be pushed or pulled.

In order to do this cross legged pose with your feet resting on the opposite thighs you have to be able to sit in a simple cross legged position and let your legs drop down so that they rest on the floor. For many Westerners this is not easy, so you can practise sitting with your back to a wall for support with your legs resting on cushions; as you exhale let your legs drop down towards the floor. When your hips begin to release you can remove the cushions and let your thighs go down to the ground.

When you can sit with both thighs well down:

1 Exhale and lift up one leg. Letting the thigh rotate outwards bring the foot to rest on the opposite thigh near the groin. The other leg stays resting on the ground.

2 Let your hips drop down as you exhale and lengthen upwards. This is half lotus pose (Ardha Padmasana)*.

3 Bring the lower leg up as you exhale and as the thigh turns outwards bring the foot up to rest on the opposite thigh as near to the groin as possible. The legs cross at the shin bones and both thighs and hips stay down.

4 Relax your shoulders and let your hands rest on your thighs. The more the hips and thighs drop the easier it is to stay in the position. At first you may not be able to stay for more than a few seconds, but with practice it will slowly become easier as you are able to 'let go' in the pose.

Remember to practise the pose with the legs crossed the other way.

Variation: You can exhale and bend forwards in this pose so that your head touches the ground in front of you. Your hips should stay down so that you lengthen in the back of the waist as you do this.

You can also twist round from this pose. Exhale, keep the hips down and turn your trunk so that one hand can reach behind your back to hold the foot that is on the opposite thigh. Keep your shoulders relaxed as you do this. The movement must come from the spine and not by pulling on the arms.

Fish pose (Matsyasana) **

This is another variation of lotus pose.

1 Lie on your back with your legs in lotus pose.
2 With your knees facing upwards, exhale and let the back of your waist touch the floor.
3 On another exhalation let your legs go down towards the floor keeping the back of your waist as long as possible. The movement should be in your hip joints. Your waist is bound to curve up a little bit but keep this movement to a minimum. Your front hip bones should come towards your waist and your tailbone should lengthen away from it.

4 Stay for several minutes breathing quietly.

5 Then repeat the pose with the legs crossed the other way round.

At the beginning it may be difficult to drop the legs right down to touch the ground. If this is the case, rest them on a cushion so that they can relax as you exhale.

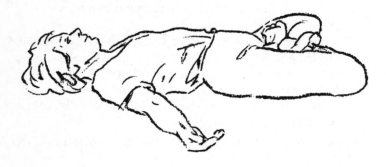

Bound lotus (Baddha Padmasana) ***

1 Sit in lotus pose with the left foot uppermost.
2 Keep your weight on both hips so that you can grow tall as you cross your arms behind your back.

3 Hold your right foot with your right hand and your left foot with your left hand.
4 Keep the back of your waist long and your chin in.
5 Repeat on the other side.

Cow pose (Gomukhasana) **

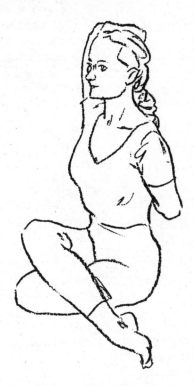

1 Sit with your thighs crossed over each other.
2 Sitting tall exhale and drop one arm down and bend the elbow, turning it so the hand is behind your back with the palm facing outwards, the fingers resting along your upper spine pointing towards your neck.
3 Raise the other arm and, bending the elbow, drop the hand behind your head to clasp the other hand behind your back. Keep the top elbow back behind your head and keep your neck straight.
4 Change over and do the other side.

Beginners should practise the arm movements only when standing in mountain pose (see page 125, Chapter 7).

Sage's twist (Marichyasana) **

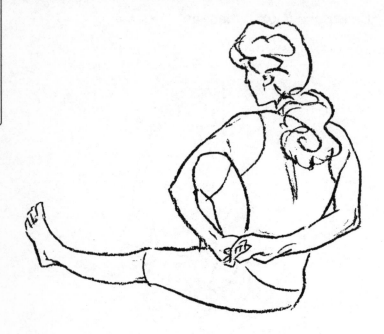

1 Sit as for Sage's pose on page 55 with one leg straight and the other leg bent up with the foot on the floor close to the buttock.
2 Sit tall, dropping the pelvis and letting your back grow upwards. Exhale and turn towards your bent leg.
3 Keeping your straight leg down, lengthen the back of your waist until your shoulders are outside your bent thigh.
4 Dropping the elbow that is closest to your thigh turn your arm and, bending the elbow, entwine the arm round your bent leg,
5 Exhaling, let the other arm reach behind your back so that your hands can clasp behind you.

6 Continue to drop your hips and straighten upwards each time you exhale, letting your hands come closer together. The more your upper back straightens the easier this will be.

Then repeat the pose on the other side.

Caution: This movement must come from the spine as it lengthens and turns. Don't push your arm against your knee, or lever yourself into the position. Go slowly – it may take time before you can catch your hands together. The ease with which you will be able to do these twisting movements with the hands held behind the back depends to some extent on bodily proportions.

Sage's twist 2 (Ardha Matsyendrasana) **

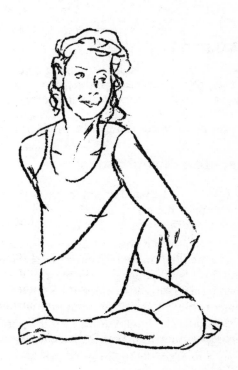

1 Sitting on the floor with your left leg folded as in half bound angle pose lift your hips up and sit on the arch of your left foot.

2 Cross the right leg over your left thigh.

3 Turn to the right until your left shoulder is outside the right thigh.

4 Drop your left arm so that the elbow nearly touches the ground then turn your arm so that the elbow can bend around your folded leg.

5 Exhale and take your right arm behind your back so that you can clasp your hands behind your back.

6 As you stay in the pose continue to lengthen upwards with each exhalation bringing the hands closer together as you sit tall. Then repeat the pose on the other side.

Backbends

In backbends there is a tendency to exaggerate the inward curve at the back of the waist and shorten the spine. To avoid this, allow yourself plenty of time to understand the movement of the spine with the breath in the simple locust pose before you attempt the poses where you use the hands or feet.

Locust pose (Salabhasana) *

1 Lie prone and let yourself sink down as you exhale. Feel the wave of the breath elongate you as your abdomen comes in towards the spine at the end of the exhalation.

2 Come up into the pose letting your upper body lift at the very end of the exhalation when the abdomen is in and there is a tightening of the muscles beneath the sitting bones. This grip under the sitting bones will anchor the pelvis down and allow the waist to lengthen so that you will lift into the pose without a feeling of compression at the back of the waist.

3 Keep your chin slightly in so that the back of the neck stays long and relaxed. Your legs should stay down on the ground.

Come down and lie on your back and hug your knees to your chest.

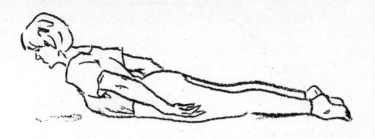

Upwards bow pose (Urdhva Dhanurasana) **

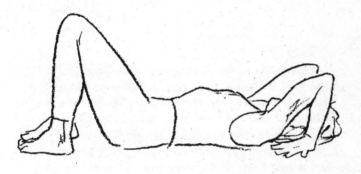

The bow bends because the bowstring pulls on each end of it evenly. In this pose the hands and feet are pulled down into the ground by gravity so that the spine can lengthen as it bends. Done like this there is a great freedom for the body to release and move. It is the exact opposite of 'pushing' up and contracting the back of the waist and neck.

1 Lie on your back with your feet parallel and close to your hips. Take your arms over your head and place your hands each side of your head with the fingers pointing back towards your feet.

2 Take time in this position, so that with each exhalation you can feel the back of your waist go down to the floor as your abdomen goes in, and let your wrists and heels go down.

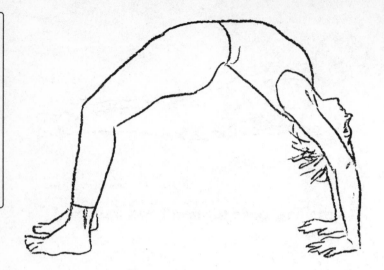

3 Come up into the pose at the very end of an exhalation when the back is very long and flat. Your hands and feet stay earthed and there should be no feeling of compression at the back of the waist.

4 As you stay in the pose the inhalation will slightly lift you up and the outbreath will allow you to earth your hands and feet, and to lengthen. Keep your chin slightly in so that the back of your neck stays long.

5 You can remain in this pose as long as you can continue to free the spine with each breath, then come down and hug your knees to your chest.

Cobra pose (Bhujangasana) **

The movement in this pose comes from the spine as in locust pose. Snakes do not have arms so do not push yourself up into the pose.

1 Lie prone with your hands at each side of your chest.

2 Come up into the pose letting your body lift with the end of the exhalation so that the pelvis is anchored down by the muscles under the sitting bones. Drop your wrists and the backs of your thighs down.

3 Keep your elbows bent and your chin slightly in.

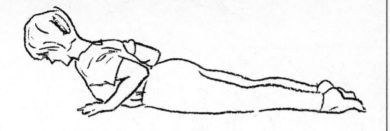

4 Don't straighten your arms and push into the back of the waist, but with each exhalation let the hands drop down as the spine bends back with the breath. For some people this means that the arms will eventually straighten, but this depends on flexibility as well as bodily proportions.

5 Come down and roll on your back and hug your knees to your chest.

This is not a difficult pose, but it needs patience not to go too far too soon without understanding the basic movement.

Squatting poses

Garland pose (Malasana) *

Some people find squatting with their heels down hard. There are various ways you can practise doing this at the beginning.

1 You can stand in mountain pose and keeping your heels down let your knees bend as you fold down into a squat; or

2 You can start in the standing forward bend, and keeping your heels down bend your knees while your trunk stays forwards as you fold in the hips; or

3 You can start in child pose so that you have a good bend in the hips and then tucking your toes under your heels use your hands to push yourself back so that your heels are on the floor. Be careful with your knees; they should point in the same direction as your feet so as not to pull them into an unnatural angle that might strain the joint.

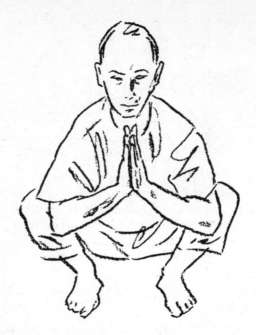

4 When you are folded down in the squat let your hips and heels go down so that your trunk goes forwards between your thighs.

5 Let your elbows drop towards the floor. If you fold forwards far enough you can take your arms out and round your legs to clasp them behind your back. This depends to some extent on bodily proportions.

Crane pose (Bakasana) **

6 From garland pose, bend your arms and tuck your elbows back behind your knees and put your hands on the floor with the fingers pointing straight in front of you.

7 As you exhale and pull your abdomen in, transfer your weight onto your hands, straightening your arms. Your feet will come onto the toes and then off the floor. Your elbows come forwards over the wrists as the arms straighten.

8 Your back curves as your abdomen tightens and your thighs grip inwards. Keep your heels tucked up near your buttocks. Come down and relax in child pose.

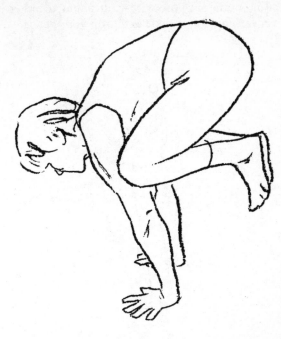

Caution: This pose can tighten the neck and shoulders; do shoulderstand later in your practice to counteract this. If you are afraid of collapsing on your face put a cushion in front of you.

Salute to the Sun (Surya Namaskar) *

This sequence is a prayer of movement and breath, of concentration and symmetry. Traditionally it is done twelve times, once for each month of the year, and it is made up of twelve positions. At the centre is a prostration where eight parts of the body touch the ground: the two hands, two knees, two feet, the chest and the chin.

The sequence can either be done with the rhythm of the inhalation and exhalation as indicated below or it can be practised more slowly exhaling with each movement and holding the positions for several breaths.

Caution: This sun prayer is not as easy as it looks. You should practise the positions individually and understand them before putting them together into the sequence. If you suffer from high blood pressure or certain eye problems, you should seek medical advice before attempting it, (see Chapter 7 for more information).

1 Stand in mountain pose with your palms together in the prayer position, exhale and drop your hands.

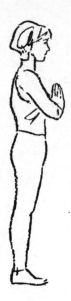

2 Raise your hands above your head; as they come up you will be inhaling.

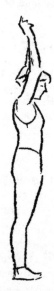

3 Exhale and go into standing forward bend; your hands should be touching the floor shoulder width apart.

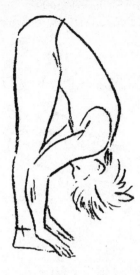

4 As you come to the end of the exhalation take your right leg back with the knee on the floor. The left heel stays down as the leg bends and you lengthen upwards with the trunk as you inhale, letting your hips drop down.

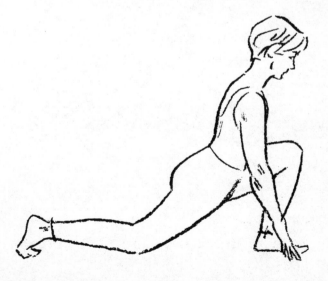

5 Holding your breath, take the left foot back to join the right and straighten the legs. Your feet should be hip width apart. Your shoulders should stay over the wrists, with arms vertical, toes tucked under.

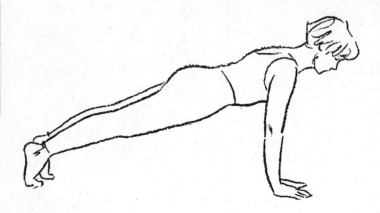

6 Exhale and bend your knees and elbows so that your toes, knees, chest, chin and hands touch the floor.

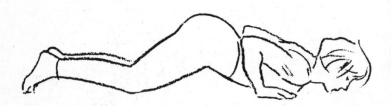

7 At the end of the exhalation tighten under your sitting bones and slide forwards coming into cobra pose; as you come to the end of this you will be inhaling.

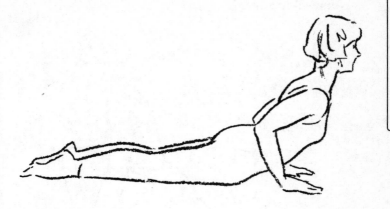

8 Exhale and go into dog pose 1.

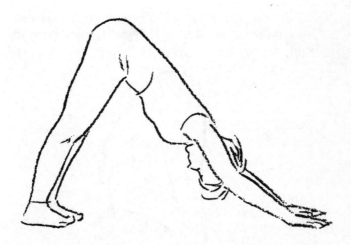

9 At the end of the exhalation swing the right leg forwards to its original position with the heel down. The left knee goes down on the floor with the foot turned under. As your hips drop and you lengthen upward you will be inhaling.

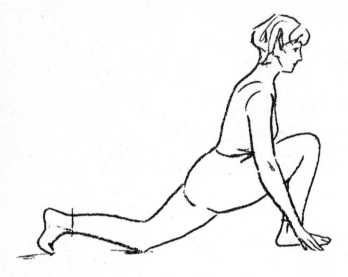

10 Exhale and bring the left leg back to its original position, straighten the legs into the standing forward bend.

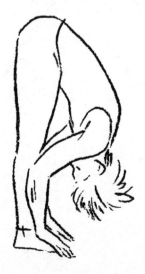

11 At the end of the exhalation let your heels go down and come up into mountain pose with your arms raised above your head. As your arms come up you will be inhaling.

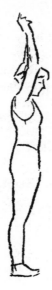

12 Exhale and resume your original position.

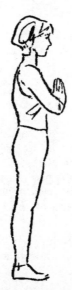

When you repeat the sequence take the left leg back at the beginning and forwards at the end to get an even stretch.

Variation: At the beginning you can practise a simplified version of the sequence, as follows, after position 4 where you have one leg back.

5 Take the other leg back and exhale as you fold into Child pose (see page 51).
6 Rest while you breathe in and then
7 exhale as you go into dog pose 1 and continue the sequence from position 9.

Relaxation poses

Recuperation pose (Supta Vajrasana) *

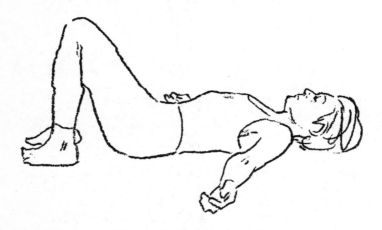

Lie on your back with your knees bent up and your feet near your buttocks. Ensure you are lying straight with your arms equidistant from your sides. As you exhale let your weight drop into the floor. Stay in this pose for two or three minutes so that the strong muscles at the back of your waist can let go, then let your legs stretch out with an exhalation so that you are lying flat in the corpse pose.

As you stretch your legs out your waist will curve up a little. If this makes the pose uncomfortable stay with the knees bent up slightly longer

Corpse pose (Savasana) *

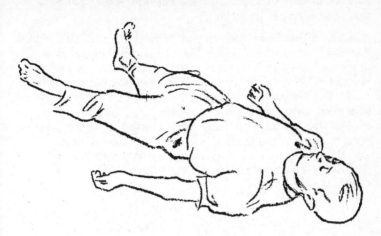

Corpse pose (Savasana) is the culmination of Yoga Asanas and should be done at the end of every practice session. Although it appears simplicity itself it is the hardest pose to practise; in this pose there is no movement to occupy your thoughts and lying completely still it is difficult to keep the mind quiet and centred in tune with the stillness of the body. To really relax and be still, not only in the body but also in the restless mind, requires stability and also courage; as we relax we sometimes have to face our inner fears, to relax our guard and face reality, and few people really wish to do that. This is why corpse pose, which is where we glimpse the beginnings of meditation, is so difficult. If your thoughts drift off into day-dreaming and your mind starts chattering to itself these distractions will cause physical tensions that disturb relaxation as well as inner peace and silence. As in all other Asanas you should follow the exhaling breath, whose gentle rhythm undoes the tension of the muscles and puts you in touch with the pull of gravity that lets us rest down on the ground if we allow ourselves to surrender to it. This focus on the breath is a way of stillness for the body and silence for the mind.

You should stay in this pose for at least ten minutes.

Caution: If the back of the neck arches so that your head tips backwards with the chin up, put a cushion under your head so that your neck can lengthen.

When you first learn Asanas and Pranayama it is a little like learning a language. You stumble over the new alphabet of the postures, learning where your arms and legs should go, when to breathe, piecing the 'letters' of the Asanas together slowly until gradually they start to fit together and you begin to make sense of it. You may still be a long way from realizing the poetry of the postures, when your body relaxes with the breath and the pose happens without effort on your part, but it starts to be interesting and fun to spring clean and retune your body each day, and to feel good after your practice.

04

Pranayama

In this chapter you will learn:
- the basic Pranayama techniques
- sitting poses for Pranayama
- about the breath as a focus for concentration.

Yoga is a thread of different strands. Asana is one strand, Pranayama is another and so is Meditation. Asanas are a way of preparing for Pranayama as they tune the body rather as a musician tunes an instrument. Pranayama tunes the body at a finer level and also calms the mind so that both body and mind become 'one-pointed' (eka gratha), which is the state needed for the practice of meditation.

Asanas balance and refine the physical body, while Pranayama balances and channels the energy that sustains life (prana). It is because of this that many warnings have been given about approaching the practice of Pranayama before having a good understanding of Yoga through Asanas and without a competent teacher. Asanas incorrectly practised might pull muscles or cause physical damage that can be easily recognized and dealt with. Pranayama, which causes changes in bodily systems and rhythms of the mind of which we are not usually consciously aware, has to be undertaken with a certain amount of caution. The golden rule is that breathing exercises should never be done with any feeling of strain or force; effort or the anxiety to achieve only results in restriction and shortness of breath which clouds the mind and may build up our sense of ego.

The breath is the pathway from the physical to the psychological and from the conscious to the unconscious. As we unlock the secrets of the body with the Asanas and old patterns of movement relax and change, so also with Pranayama there is a rebalancing at a more subtle level.

The link between the body and the mind is the breath. Rapid shallow breathing can make us anxious, drawing the breath in sharply can increase aggression. How we breathe affects the mind and our mental state is reflected in our breathing patterns. The breath is also the natural way in which we unconsciously release tension and restore energy. Both sighing and yawning are examples of involuntary therapeutic breathing.

Just as in Asanas, where the most simple poses are the most difficult with the most complicated twist or stretch merely being a means of adjusting the body so that you can sit or stand simply in harmony with the universe, so it is in Pranayama, where even the most elaborate techniques are but a way of helping you to learn to breathe slowly, simply and regularly in order to quieten the mind and bring peace and clarity. Therefore the practice of the various techniques is only appropriate when they release tensions and make concentration easier. If any technique makes you anxious or uncomfortable, or you feel strained, then this is not the right moment for you to practise it.

Preparation for Pranayama

As well as practising Asanas to prepare for Pranayama, the Hatha Yoga writings recommend Kriyas (cleansing processes), Bandhas (locks) and Mudras (seals). These help detoxify and strengthen the body.

Kriyas

These are ways of cleansing and purifying the body. They were primarily intended as a means of curing sickness: the *Hatha Yoga Pradipika* says they are for 'the flabby and phlegmatic'. Asanas and Pranayama are in themselves therapeutic but the Kriyas are more invasive techniques which can disturb the balance of a healthy body and should not be undertaken without medical advice.

1 Dhauti: Swallowing a length of cloth and regurgitating it to cleanse the stomach.

2 Vasti: Washing out the intestines by drawing up water through the rectum.

3 Neti: Cleansing the nasal passages with water or by the use of a thread.

4 Nauli: Moving the rectus abdominis muscles in a churning action to stimulate the internal organs. This is done with Uddiyana Bandha (page 83) and must be taught by a Guru.

5 Trataka: Gazing at a fixed point until the eyes water.

6 Kapalabhati: This is a preparatory exercise before practising Pranayama. It is a series of short quick exhalations with the abdomen pulled back towards the spine and then released, so causing a short involuntary inhalation. The action of the abdominal muscle helps to extend the curve at the back of the waist causing the hips to drop and the sitting position to become grounded, with the shoulders relaxed. This is an excellent lesson in how to sit and is the key to all Yoga breathing. Healthy people with good posture can practise this, but it should not be attempted by pregnant women or those suffering from prolapse. People with heart or lung problems, high blood pressure or eye disorders should seek medical advice before practising it.

Method

- Sit on your heels in thunderbolt pose (page 50) or in lotus (page 58) or half lotus (page 56).
- Inhale normally letting your abdomen relax a little.
- Exhale quickly and lightly pulling the abdomen in sharply and then immediately relaxing it again. This means that you will inhale passively as your abdomen lets go.
- Repeat by exhaling quickly as before, pulling the abdomen in and relaxing it. Once you have learned this movement and the abdominal muscles are trained so that they can contract and relax easily, you can do up to 60 quick exhalations at a stretch, at the rate of about one a second.
- The last exhalation pulls the abdomen far in; then it is released slowly for a calm, steady, passive inhalation.

This process can be repeated up to three times. How easy this is at first will depend on your normal breathing pattern; it may take some time to synchronise the pulling in of the abdomen with the outbreath. Others will find this easy. Start with ten exhalations; this will be ample as it takes practice to make the quick exhalations light, rhythmical and even. Gradually increase the number to 60.

Bandhas

Pranayama has to be practised with the aid of bandhas (locks) and mudras (seals). The action of breathing changes the pressures in the abdominal and thoracic cavities. In deep breathing these changes are more extreme than in normal everyday respiration. Bandhas are locks or holds that ensure that the pressure is used properly and no damage is done to the delicate tissues of the body. They also help ensure an elongation of the spinal curves and promote a good sitting position. Asanas help develop a good sitting posture so that the Bandhas work naturally as you breathe; deep breathing at first should be done gradually so that you can feel how your lungs work and how your spine aligns itself with the muscular action of the bandhas coming into play as the breathing deepens. You should go gently and never, ever, force the breathing. If you are in any doubt ask the guidance of a qualified teacher.

There are five principal 'airs', which constitute the vital energy, Prana, within the body. With the use of the bandhas the downwards moving 'apana', which is usually situated in the perineum, is united with the 'prana', which is in the heart. The vital energy is thus conserved and can be redirected.

Moolabandha

Sit with your pelvis straight. At the end of an exhalation, when the lower abdomen draws in towards the spine, the pelvic floor (the sheet of muscle underneath the trunk which contains the anus) should slightly tighten and lift so that there is no downward pressure from the internal organs above it. This tightening and lifting of the pelvic floor together with the contraction of the abdominal muscles below the navel is the action of the Moolabandha.

Jalandhara Bandha

This controls the pressure at the top of the thoracic cavity and also helps to elongate the spine as it straightens the neck. It can also exert pressure on the carotoid arteries at the side of the neck which control the blood supply to the brain. To form the Jalandhara Bandha, let your neck lengthen as the back of your skull moves upwards and the chin draws in level with the notch in between the collar bones at the front of the neck, so there is a slight pressure at the sides of your jaw. Keep your eyes relaxed and looking downwards. This not only controls the pressure when you hold your breath, but it ensures that the whole of the spine lengthens from the sacrum to the top of the neck where it enters the skull. This lengthening of the neck and chin lock are developed through the practice of shoulderstand (Sarvangasana, page 39).

Uddiyana Bandha

This movement controls the abdominal muscles, which form the front wall of the trunk. The strength of these muscles balances with the curve of the lumbar spine at the waist, which lengthens as the abdominal muscles contract. The contraction of the abdomen pushes the internal organs back towards the spine and upwards towards the diaphragm, increasing the pressure in the thoracic cavity so that more air than normal is expelled. The following inhalation will correspondingly be deeper.

At the end of each exhalation, this Bandha will happen by itself if you are sitting straight so that your spine can stretch upwards as the sitting bones go down. You can also feel this movement in headstand (Sirsasana) because the inverted posture reverses the normal pull of gravity on the diaphragm and abdominal muscles. If the headstand is straight you will feel the area between the pubic bone and the front ribs become hollow at the end of the outbreath. Uddiyana Bandha can also be practised as a separate exercise to develop the strength of the abdominal muscles.

- Stand with your knees slightly bent and your weight on your heels and feet parallel and slightly apart.
- Keeping your back long and your shoulders relaxed put your hands on your knees.
- The back of your neck should be long and your chin should be in (Jalandhara Bandha, page 83).
- Exhale fully so that your abdomen goes in and your navel moves back towards your spine.
- Holding the breath out, pull the abdomen further in and lift the navel upwards towards your diaphragm. The internal organs and the wall of the abdomen should be sucked back towards the spine and there should be a hollow from the pubic bone to the lower border of the ribs. Slowly relax your grip on the abdominal muscles as you breathe in. This exercise can also be practised in the lotus pose.

Caution: This exercise should not be attempted by anyone with high blood pressure, heart problems, detached retina, circulatory or breathing problems or during pregnancy.

Asanas that help develop the action of the Bandhas

Dog pose with the head down (Svanasana, page 34)

In dog pose 1 the trunk is slanting downwards with the hips uppermost. In this position the Moolabandha forms naturally as you exhale and pull in the lower abdomen; the pelvic floor will be drawn inwards and down with the force of gravity. The same applies to the Uddiyana Bandha; as the abdomen and solar plexus are drawn inwards the internal organs move towards the diaphragm on the exhalation. The weight of your head, as it hangs down, allows the back of the neck to lengthen and the chin to draw slightly inwards in the Jalandhara Bandha. In this pose the Bandhas form passively, whereas when you are sitting or standing they are done actively using muscular strength as in the following pose.

Maha Mudra

Sit with the left leg stretched out in front of you and the right leg folded so that the foot is close to the inside of the left thigh. The heel should touch the pubic bone and the thighs should be at right angles. Keeping your sitting bones down and your spine long, hold your left foot with with your right hand (if this is difficult loop a belt round your foot and hold that). Exhale and let the pelvis and right thigh drop and the spine straighten upwards. The pelvic floor should tighten and the abdomen draw inwards. As the waist and neck lengthen the chin also draws inwards. There should be maximum distance between the sitting bones and the back of the skull. Inhale, relaxing the abdomen and then repeat the position on the other side with the right leg straight.

Mudras

In some of the old texts these are listed as being the same as Bandhas, but they serve a slightly different function as they close or complete circuits of energy without having a direct effect on the spine, or control of the pressure in the bodily cavities. They are also said to bring stability and quietness as the body becomes 'centred'.

Kerachi Mudra

This is used in some Pranayama techniques. Turn your tongue back so that its underside touches the roof of your mouth. With the tongue in this position, your head finds the right balance at the top of the neck. It is difficult to poke the chin too far forwards when the tongue is tucked back.

Jnana Mudra

Touch the tip of your thumb to the tip of your index finger. This symbolizes the union of the individual soul with the Infinite. Sometimes this position of the hands is used in Pranayama, but used wrongly it merely causes tension in the shoulders, which can interfere with the breathing.

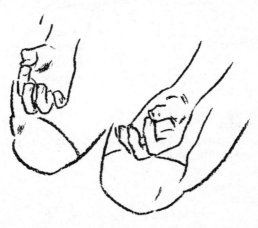

Sanmukhi Mudra

Sit in lotus pose (page 58), or half lotus pose, and close your eyes. Put your hands gently over your face with your thumbs closing your ears and the soft undersides of the fingers spread out so that the index fingers are on the eyebrows, the middle fingers just below your eyes, the ring fingers at the corners of the nostrils and the little fingers at the corners of the mouth. As you exhale the pressure of the fingers allows the centre of the face to widen, the frowning lines between the eyebrows to relax, the corners of the mouth to release any tension and your face feels quiet and calm.

Caution: Never press directly on the eyeballs.

A similar effect can be obtained when you are lying in corpse pose (Savasana, page 77) by putting a small bag (30 × 10 cm) filled with a little rice over your eyes. The rice will fall towards each end of the bag helping the eyes and face to relax and widen. Do not make the bag too full as there should be no heavy direct pressure on the eyeballs.

People with eye problems must ask a qualified medical doctor before using this technique.

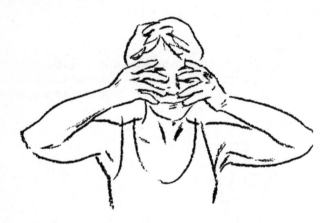

Asvini Mudra

Closing the anal sphincter muscle. This is part of the Moolabandha movement.

The action of breathing

The main muscle of respiration is the diaphragm, which lies across the trunk separating the thorax from the abdomen. It is attached to the bottom of the sternum (breastbone) and to the lower borders of the ribcage; this means that it is higher in the front than at the back, where it ends in two long muscles that anchor it to the inside of the lumbar spine almost at the level of the hips. This slanting position means that the lungs that lie above it are longer at the back than in the front.

The diaphragm is always domed upwards, rather like an open umbrella with no handle. As you inhale it contracts in the centre and slightly flattens expanding the volume of the chest lengthways, thus reducing the pressure in the lungs so that air is sucked into them through the windpipe. On exhalation the diaphragm relaxes and moves up again so that the volume in the chest decreases, the pressure within the lungs increases and the air is sucked out again. The chest also expands widthways because on inhalation the descent of the diaphragm is eventually stopped by the resistance of the liver and stomach, which lie beneath it. As it continues to contract at the centre it now pulls the lower ribs upwards and the ribcage expands outwards with the help of the intercostal muscles. For this action to work

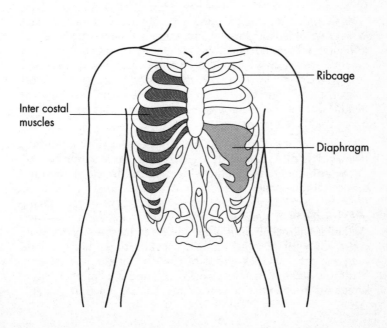

efficiently there has to be a rhythmical, reciprocal action between the diaphragm and the abdominal muscles; if the abdominal muscles are rigid and unyielding the descent of the diaphragm is blocked too soon and the chest pushes out arching the spine at the waist and restricting the back of the lungs as the diaphragm continues to contract.

Asanas practised using the breath should ensure that the muscles work properly. When you sit for Pranayama or meditation you have to choose a position where the curves of your spine can balance properly and the diaphragm and lungs can function efficiently.

Sitting positions for Pranayama

You have to sit with the pelvis straight and your two sitting bones firmly down on the floor so that your spine is free to balance itself easily in its four elongating curves. As you sit your head should find its own point of balance at the top of the neck in accordance with the pull of gravity on the pelvis and the release of the spine as it adjusts and readjusts as you inhale and exhale. For this to happen the position has to be stable at the base and relaxed and free at the top. Your hands should rest on your knees so that your arms can relax downwards away from your shoulders leaving the upper part of your chest unrestricted. When first practising Pranayama, there is sometimes a tendency to tighten the shoulders and lift the elbows on inhalation. When inhaling, your elbows should drop and your palms stay relaxed. Sitting well means that the respiratory muscles can work properly, and that the spine can balance remaining tall and flexible so that the position can be held for a long time without becoming fixed or rigid.

The position of the pelvis, the base of the pose, is all important. If the pelvis tilts backwards the natural incurve at the back of the waist bulges back and the whole spine is dragged backwards into a stooping position, which restricts the front of the chest. If the pelvis is tilted too far forwards the incurve of the waist is exaggerated and there is a downward pressure on the lower abdomen and pelvic floor. The muscles at the back of the waist contract to pull the trunk straight, blocking the expansion of the lungs at the back. In either of these incorrect positions the breathing action is made more difficult and the Bandhas, which safeguard the practice of Pranayama, cannot function.

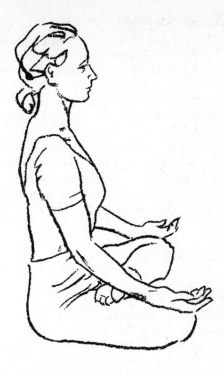

The best position for sitting with the pelvis straight is lotus pose (Padmasana, page 58) as here the thighs rest on the ground held by the feet. The position is grounded and secure with the hips well down and the spine free.

Caution: If you are flexible enough to use lotus pose for Pranayama or Meditation remember to use the right leg first as you cross your legs one day and the left leg first the next day. If you always cross the legs the same way you risk developing an uneven movement in the hips.

Thunderbolt pose (Vajrasana, page 50) also allows the pelvis to sit straight. The problem here is that you tend to get pins and needles in the feet. Also for some people, the feet and knees are too stiff for this to be comfortable. To help with this you can put a rolled towel under your feet and/or sit with a cushion placed over your heels.

Caution: Be sure that your feet are straight so that your sitting bones are evenly supported so that you have a firm base on which to sit.

Pranayama in a chair

You can also practise Pranayama and meditation sitting in a chair. Be sure that your pelvis is straight and do not lean against the back of the chair as your spine must be erect and able to balance itself as you breathe. If the chair is too low to allow your thighs to rest horizontally, put a cushion on the seat; if it is too high for your feet to rest comfortably on the floor, put a book beneath them.

Hero pose (Virasana) and bound angle pose (Baddha Konasana) tend to tilt the pelvis too far backwards unless you are very flexible in the hips. It will therefore be difficult for the average person to maintain these poses for any length of time; equally the sitting poses with straight legs will also be unsuitable.

Simple breathing

Deep breathing (Ujayii)

Sit in lotus pose (Padmasana, page 58) or on your heels (Vajrasana, page 50). Exhale slowly letting the abdomen draw in towards the spine. As this happens the back of the waist will extend and your hips will drop. Relax your shoulders so that your head balances effortlessly at the top of the neck as your spine lengthens upwards. At the end of the exhalation, be still and allow the breath to come in passively. Keep your hips down so that the pose stays grounded. With the hips down the spine is free to align naturally as the lungs fill. Do not attempt to take the breath in or lift the chest as this will merely shorten the back of the body and interfere with the action of the diaphragm.

Continue breathing like this. The spine will lengthen upwards as you exhale, the hips will drop and your shoulders will relax. Your body should find its own balance of perfect equilibrium so that the breathing becomes a continual unconscious rhythmical adjustment of the spine in accordance with the pull of gravity. This breathing teaches the perfect sitting posture just as the perfect sitting posture teaches us to breathe.

As your breathing becomes steady count the seconds so that the inhalation and exhalation become equal and the flow of the breath smooth and even. Start with a count of four seconds; you will find that with practice and concentration the length of your breaths will extend without effort.

If you are worried or upset, or strain to lengthen the breath forcefully, your breathing will become shorter and uneven. With regular practice this gentle slow deep breathing will become second nature, a way of steadying and centring yourself that can be used at times of stress as well as being part of a daily routine.

Pranayama techniques that change the ratio of inhalation and exhalation

Interval breathing (Viloma)

Sit in Lotus Pose (Padmasana, page 58) or on your heels (Vajrasana, page 50).

Interval breathing on the inhalation

Exhale as in Ujayii. Relax and let the hips drop, start to inhale passively, pause then inhale further, pause, inhale completely then pause and exhale as in Ujayii. Repeat the inhalation with the pauses keeping the length and number of pauses even.

Interval breathing on the exhalation

Exhale as in Ujayii then inhale passively as in Ujayii. At the end of the inhalation pause, exhale a little and pause, exhale a little further and pause again, exhale fully and then inhale passively. Repeat the exhalation with the pauses keeping the length and number of pauses even.

Caution: Do not pause at the very end of the exhalation as this can make you feel short of breath.

When you pause drop your hips and let the spine lengthen upwards. You should feel grounded with the spine and shoulders free. The pauses are moments of perfect silence, stillness and equilibrium. The pauses and intervals of breathing should be even in length. Start with one second of inhalation and one second's pause, then increase this to two seconds. You can also increase the number of pauses. When these two techniques are familiar you can practise them together, pausing on the inhalation and the exhalation.

Caution: Be sure that you pause completely. It is easy to exhale slightly when pausing on the inhalation and vice versa. Interval breathing is a way of learning to extend the length of the inhalation or exhalation, and it introduces a way of holding the breath without a feeling of restriction or tension. Make yourself familiar with this technique before trying to hold the breath.

Holding the breath (Kumbaka)

This is a cessation of breathing that crystallizes, for a matter of seconds, the moving spiral of the breath that brings you to a point of balance at the end of the inhalation or exhalation. Concentration, stillness and silence are not tests of endurance but ways to integration; Kumbaka must be practised with this in mind. The stopping of the breath should bring a sense of calmness and clarity not a feeling of tension and suffocation. Individual capacity will vary enormously and the timing of the retention of the breath will lengthen naturally with practice. It must never be forced.

Method

In this technique, the exhalation should be twice the length of the inhalation. For example, if the inhalation is five seconds then the exhalation will be ten seconds. First then, you need to practise breathing as in Ujayii with this one to two ratio.

Inhale for five seconds and then stop the breath. As you do this drop your hips and relax your shoulders so that your spine can grow tall. There should be a feeling of lightness and also complete stability; you retain the breath by allowing it freedom. The longer your spine and the looser your shoulders, the longer you will be able to hold the breath. Keep your hands passive – there is a tendency to tighten them when you retain the breath.

Stay still and silent for five seconds and then exhale for ten seconds. When this comes easily, increase the duration of the retention so that the ratio is five seconds inhalation, ten seconds retention and ten seconds exhalation. Later you can practise five seconds inhalation, fifteen seconds retention and ten seconds exhalation. This ratio of 1, 3, 2, should be maintained for any increase in the length of retention.

Pranayama techniques where the breath is channelled through different nostrils

In Hatha Yoga the principal nadis – the Pingala which carries the solar energy Ha and the Ida which carries the lunar energy THA – pass through the right and left nostrils respectively. This series of exercises where the breath is controlled by the pressure of the fingers on the nostrils aims to balance these energies. They are not suitable for beginners because the use of the hands can disturb the alignment and stability of the sitting position. They can also cause tension in the shoulders if they are practised too soon.

How to use the fingers to close the nostrils

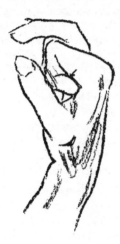

1 Sit in lotus pose or sit on your heels.
2 Bring your right hand towards your nose. Your head must stay in line with your spine and not bend forwards towards your hand.
3 Keep your shoulders relaxed and your wrist loose.
4 Your fingers should touch your nose where the hard bone meets the cartilage, about half way down the side of the nose. Very little pressure here will close the channel.
5 Keep your wrist up so that the fingers are horizontal; they must not pull downwards.
6 The tip of your right thumb closes the right nostril; the tips of the ring and little finger held together close the left nostril. The other two fingers are folded down in the centre of the palm and held under the base of the thumb bone.
7 Take care that the right hand does not pull your head over to the right as you practise. To avoid this at first you can get the feeling of the technique by using the

hands alternately and closing the nostrils with the tips of the index fingers, keeping the position of the head centred. Later use the right hand as instructed above.

Alternate nostril breathing (Nadi Sodhana)

In this exercise the inhalation and exhalation use alternate channels which change when the lungs are full. The purpose of this is to cleanse the nadis.

- Start by inhaling through both nostrils, then close the left nostril and exhale and inhale through the right.
- Close the right nostril, release the left nostril and exhale and inhale through the left.
- Close the left nostril, release the right nostril and exhale and inhale through the right.
- Continue like this changing the channels after each inhalation.
- Finish by exhaling through the right nostril.

The length of the breaths should be even and the flow of the air steady. To ensure this, the fingers can be used to regulate the size of the aperture and the the flow of the breath on the side through which you are breathing. This applies to all the following alternate nostril breathing techniques.

Alternate nostril exhalation (Anuloma)

Here the inhalation is always through both nostrils and the exhalation is through the right nostril and then on the next breath through the left nostril and then on the right again on the following exhalation.

Alternate nostril inhalation (Pratiloma)

The exhalation is always through both nostrils and the inhalation is through the right nostril and then on the next breath through the left nostril.

Inhalation through the sun channel (Surya Bhedana)

The pingala nadi ends at the right nostril. This Pranayama warms the body as the inhalation is done only on that side.

- Exhale through both nostrils.
- Close the left nostril and inhale through the right.
- Close the right nostril, release the left and exhale.
- Continue with all inhalations through the right and all exhalations through the left.
- Finish by inhaling and exhaling through both nostrils.

Inhalation through the moon channel (Chandra Bedana)

- Exhale through both nostrils.
- Close the right nostril and inhale through the left.
- Close the left nostril and release the right and exhale.
- Continue with all inhalations on the left side and all exhalations on the right. This inhaling through the left nostril, which is the path of Ida the moon channel, cools the body.

Techniques that use the mouth

Cooling breath (Sitali)

This exercise uses the tongue with the inhalation through the mouth. It releases tension in the neck and head. Inhaling along the tongue entails sucking in saliva which is swallowed so it is considered to be a good Pranayama to practise in hot weather as it cools you down and reduces thirst. Sit in lotus pose or sit on your heels, then commence the breathing cycle.

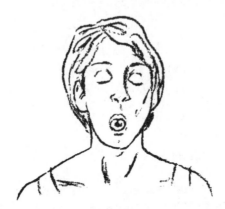

- Sit tall with your sitting bones down and your shoulders relaxed.
- Purse your lips to make an O.
- Stick out your tongue curling the outer edges inwards so that it makes a tube.
- Throw your head back as far as you can and, stretching your tongue out as much as possible, suck the air in through your mouth along your tongue. The tongue should stretch out as you do this and you should feel it elongating from under your jaw and also at the sides of your neck.

- At the end of the inhalation curl your tongue back and swallow any saliva that has collected in your mouth.
- Lift your head and let your neck straighten by bringing in your chin (Jalandhara Bandha, page 83). Then exhale slowly through your nose.
- The hips should drop and the back of the skull moves upwards as the spine straightens.
- Repeat the cycle.

Lion breath

This exercise uses the tongue on the exhalation. It is a strong, powerful cleansing breath that also opens the palms of the hands and the soles of the feet and directs the eyes upwards. It releases a lot of tension round the head and neck and is said to be excellent for a sore throat or cold.

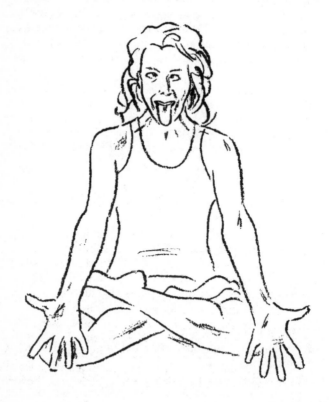

- Sit in a cross legged position, preferably lotus or half lotus pose.
- Inhale normally.
- Open the mouth wide and exhale strongly, stretching out your tongue so that the tip of it tries to touch your chin.
- At the same time open the palms of your hands and the soles of your feet (keep your shoulders relaxed).
- Make sure that your eyes look upwards towards the spot between your eyebrows.
- Your chin should be in (Jalandhara Bandha, page 83).
- There should be a vibration from the throat as you exhale.
- Inhale normally, and then repeat for no more than four breaths.

Exhaling with a vibration (Bramari)

This is an exhalation through the mouth that makes a buzzing sound like a bee. It starts with a vibration on the lips, but is felt internally rather than sounded externally. You should be able to feel the vibration if you put your hand on the back of your neck or head. With practice, as you lengthen the spine and sit tall with the shoulders relaxed and the hips down, you will feel the vibration in the ribcage and then down the spine. At first the vibration is hard to feel unless you buzz quite strongly like an angry bumble bee but eventually it will become quieter and more like the contented hum of honey bees on a sunny day.

- Sit in lotus pose or on your heels.
- Exhale slowly.
- Let the inhalation be very quiet, keeping your shoulders relaxed.
- Exhale through the mouth letting your lips vibrate to make a gentle buzzing sound. Keep your shoulders relaxed and drop your hips letting your spine lengthen and straighten so that you can focus the vibration down the spine as the abdomen goes in at the end of the exhalation.
- Release the abdomen and inhale. Continue.

You cannot drop the vibration down the spine unless you are sitting tall with the hips well grounded and the shoulders, hands and face passive. Any tension will block the vibration. This is an extremely calming and also cleansing technique. It is excellent for relaxing the neck and shoulders and teaching you how to sit well.

AUM

This Sanskrit word is one of the oldest sounds or vibrations used for prayer or meditation. The root sound of the vowel means wholeness and completion in other languages besides Sanskrit (Omega in Greek, for example). When pronounced correctly the sound is said to encompass all known vowel sounds and to be the vibration of creation. As well as symbolizing the differing states of consciousness (see page 3) AUM also signifies the link between the Creator and Creation, a bond like that between parent and child. AUM is this link expressed through sound.

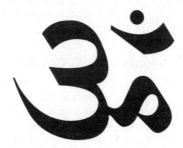

When the vibration makes a continuous mmmmmmmm you can sound AUMmmmm as you exhale. To begin with, take five seconds for the vowel and ten seconds for the vibrating mmm.

This is not a chant for others to hear, or to be done in unison. Rather, it is an interior sound that continues in a vibration, descending from the head to the base of the spine.

Breathing as a focus for concentration

Breathing is used as a way of focusing the mind for meditation in all major world religions, although in some cases the practice has, at times, been discouraged or hidden.

The breath is a powerful medium uniting the functions of body and mind, and affects our physical and mental state. While under conscious control ultimately breathing is a function of our unconscious desire for survival. An infinitely precious thing – our gift at birth and the last thing we relinquish when we die – breathing is the concrete manifestation of the life within us, personal to each of us and yet universal.

Whichever 'way' of meditation we choose to adopt, it will eventually be integrated with our breathing; as we concentrate, our breathing patterns change and slow down. Our posture, breath and mental focus harmonise and become one.

All the exercises of Pranayama can be used as a prelude to meditation which leads us to concentrate with quiet steady breathing that focuses to a single point of awareness.

Practical reminders

1 Regular practice is very important. If you have to miss Asana practice for some reason, find time to do Pranayama.

2 Practise at the same time of day if at all possible.

3 Don't practise on a full or on a completely empty stomach. If practising early in the morning have a drink of milk beforehand.

4 Always sit with the pelvis straight and the spine and head erect. The spine should be free to adjust as you breathe, not rigid.

5 Breathe through the nose unless otherwise instructed.

6 Unless otherwise instructed, the length of the inhalation should be the same as the exhalation.

7 Practise Kapalbhati at the beginning of your practice to help you sit relaxed and stable, then do one of the exercises if this helps you to concentrate. Finally do simple Ujayii breathing.

8 **Never force or push your breathing**. Apart from anything else, that only makes it more difficult.

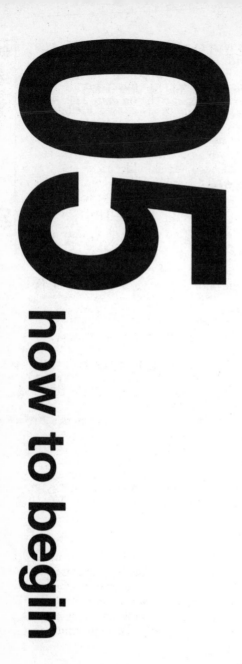

05

how to begin

In this chapter you will learn:
- how to plan your practice
- what you need
- what to do.

To learn Yoga you have to start to practise.

Where
You need a flat surface where it is warm and out of a draft. Find a space where you have enough room to lie on your back with your arms stretched out over your head.

Equipment
If the floor is at all slippery you will need a non-slip mat. You will need a rug or blanket for head and shoulderstand, and you may need a belt (pages 47, 50, 58). When you practise headstands you will need a mirror to see if you are straight. This is vital if you do not have a teacher. The mirror must go down to the floor and be perpendicular.

Clothes
Should be light and stretchy and you must have bare feet. For women a T-shirt and leggings or pants will be far more comfortable than a leotard. Have a sweater and socks to wear for Pranayama and relaxation. You should not get chilled after doing the Asanas.

When
Practising at a set time is helpful. You should not practise just after a meal when you have a full stomach, or late at night when you are tired. Choose a time when you are unlikely to be disturbed and don't answer the telephone.

How long
You don't have to devote hours and hours of your time, but you do have to practise regularly. At the beginning aim at having half an hour – 20 minutes for the Asanas, five minutes for Pranayama and five minutes for relaxation. Once a week give yourself an hour so that you can discover more about the Asanas and spend a little longer on Pranayama and relaxing.

What to practise
At the beginning keep to a set routine which allows you to stretch your body evenly in the allotted time. You can use the practice plans at the end of this chapter or do the beginner's version of the Salute to the Sun on page 76 followed by relaxation. Later you can listen to your body and vary your practice accordingly; this is not necessarily the same thing as self-indulgence.

Guidelines for planning Asana practice

1 Always start your practice with simple Asanas to allow your body to warm up gradually.

2 At the end of your practice give yourself time to quieten down with sitting Asanas before Pranayama and relaxation.

3 All the Asanas marked with one asterisk (*) can be practised by beginners and will be found in the practice plans on page 103. For most people the Asanas marked with two asterisks (**) are more difficult and should only be attempted after some months. The Asanas marked with three asterisks (***) require strength and flexibility and some years of experience.

4 Movements must vary in each practice session, backbends being followed by frontbends as 'counterposes' and energetic poses being combined with quieter more relaxing ones. Counterposes are not one extreme movement followed by another in the opposite direction; rather they are a way of bringing the body to a state of equilibrium. In Yoga the aim is to let the curves of the spine elongate, not to exaggerate them. It is to ensure this that counterposes are used.

5 Headstand is not a pose for beginners. When practised it should always be followed by shoulderstand, a calming resting pose that stretches the neck and provides a counterpose. Shoulderstand should also be practised after crane pose to elongate the neck.

6 We are all crooked to a greater or lesser extent from being right- or left-handed, or from habits that go back to childhood, from the routine movements we make at work or from the physical expression of stress. As you begin to practise Asanas you will discover where your particular stiffness is and which positions help alleviate this. Keep this in mind when planning your practice – for example if you have a stiff shoulder which makes shoulderstand a problem do a position such as cow pose (page 61) or dog pose (page 34) to release the shoulder first. In the asymmetrical poses you may find one side is easier than the other. You should of course pay more attention to the difficult side.

7 Stay alert to the fact that things change, stiff hips loosen up, crooked spines straighten, stamina improves; last year's practice may no longer be appropriate.

Practice series for beginners

Practice A

Do this series of Asanas every day for the first month.

1 Standing straight pose (page 25): This will align with the pull of gravity.

2 Triangle pose (page 31): Stretches the spine from a firm base.

3 Tree pose (page 26): To balance and centre you again.

4 Standing forward bend (page 32): Go forwards to a chair unless your hands touch the floor easily.

5 Shoulderstand (page 39): Go slowly; if difficult use a chair as on page 120.

6 Plough (page 40): Use a chair unless your feet touch the floor easily. At first do shoulderstand and plough separately. Later when you can stay longer in the poses, practise plough as a continuation of shoulderstand.

7 Supine twist (page 48): This will release any tension in your neck and shoulders after the inverted poses.

8 Sitting on the heels: For Pranayama. Five minutes. Use a cushion or blanket under your feet or heels if necessary.

9 Corpse pose (page 77): For total quiet and stillness.

Pranayama for the first month

To begin with, sit and feel what is happening when you breathe. Don't try to *do* anything, just observe the breath, letting your shoulders relax and focusing on the exhalation.

Practice B

For the second month, do this series of Asanas and Practice A on alternate days.

1 Standing straight pose.

2 Triangle pose or extended angle pose (page 31).

3 Triangle twist pose (page 32): This will rotate the spine from the hips. It is more difficult to keep grounded on the back heel, so be firm in triangle pose before you attempt this.

4 Warrior pose (page 29): This centres you as well as giving a strong elongation.

5 Eagle pose (page 28): Arms only to begin with, this will release any tension in the shoulders after warrior pose.

6   Wide astride standing pose (page 33). If difficult go forwards to a chair.

7   Shoulderstand (page 39). Stay in the pose up to five minutes.

8   Plough as a continuation of shoulderstand.

9   Supine leg stretches (page 47): These movements come easily after inverted poses.

10 Dog pose (page 34): To stretch the spine and neck after inverted poses.

11 Sitting on the heels for Pranayama.

12 Corpse pose. To relax.

Pranayama for the second month
Use the abdominal muscles as you exhale. Try a few rounds of Kapalabhati (page 81).

Practice C

For the third month, do this series of Asanas in rotation with Practice A and Practice B.

1   Recuperation pose (page 76): Let your spine lengthen with the exhalation.

2   Supine leg stretches (page 47): Concentrate on moving with the exhalation.

3   Child pose (page 51): Spine long, shoulders relaxed.

4   Dog pose (with head down): At first go from child pose into dog pose two or three times. When it is easy, do dog pose once staying in the position for several breaths. This will relax the neck and shoulders before inverted poses, (page 36).

5   Shoulderstand (page 39): You should be comfortable staying up to five minutes, then go into plough.

6   Plough: Then roll down with the legs straight.

7   Supine twist (page 48): To relax the neck and shoulders.

8   Locust pose (page 64): Extends the whole spine backwards.

9   Half bound angle pose (page 54): A forward stretching counterpose after backbends.

10 Half hero pose (page 54).

11 Sage's pose: A sitting, twisting movement that relaxes shoulders (page 55).

12 Sitting on the heels or half lotus for Pranayama (page 88).

13 Corpse pose to relax.

This series of Asanas will take a little longer than the others.

Pranayama for the third month.
Continue to practise Kapalabhati, gradually increasing the number of exhalations in each round. This will help you sit with your shoulders relaxed and your spine long with the pelvis well down. Ten exhalations in each round with deep, slow Ujayii breathing in between.

After three months' practice you will have an idea of where your strengths and weakness are and you can change your routine to suit your needs. When you feel ready to do more difficult poses you can add headstand to any of the series of Asanas, doing it before shoulderstand. (Headstand needs strong spinal muscles – a good rule is to try it only when you can stay in shoulderstand without collapsing for at least ten minutes.) You can also extend the range of the other poses.

A longer practice would take one of the following forms:

Practice D

1 Salute to the sun or standing poses.
2 Inverted poses.
3 Supine leg stretches.
4 Backbends.
5 Forward bends and sitting poses.
6 Twists, ending with a straight forward bend to centre yourself.
7 Pranayama.
8 Relaxation.

Practice E

1 Recuperation pose.
2 Supine leg stretches.
3 Inverted poses.
4 Backbends.
5 Forward bends.

6 Twists ending with a straight forward bend to centre yourself.

7 Pranayama.

8 Relax.

In Pranayama the arts of sitting and breathing go together. Kapalabhati and Ujayii (deep breathing) should be learned first. The other techniques are only valuable when they contribute to a stable sitting position and a feeling of alert inner silence and stillness.

The number of poses you practise in each category will depend on the time available to you. Quality is a great deal more important than quantity. Go slowly so that you can be observant as you practise and above all enjoy it.

Yoga is a path of liberation. One of the worst mistakes we can make is to turn it into a way of purgatory, where we beat our bodies into compliance through Asanas and Pranayama. When we do Yoga we will find that we need to discard negative and destructive habits. If we pay attention we will begin to understand the structure and meaning of the body; naturally, we discover the source of vitality and joy that is within us. The attention needed for this is love.

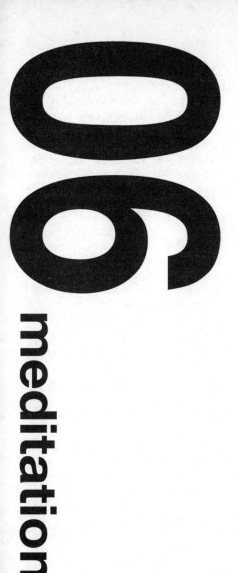

06

meditation

In this chapter you will learn:
- what Yoga meditation is
- how to practise
- different ways to start
- about problems that may arise.

Classical Yoga

The last three steps of Patanjali's Classical Yoga concern meditation. They are Dharana (Concentration), Dhyana (Meditation) and Samadhi (Illumination). Collectively they are known as Samyama – the inner path. The step that precedes these is Pratyahara, which is usually rather clumsily translated as 'withdrawal of the senses'. The practice of Yoga Asanas and Pranayama centres your attention on what you are doing, focusing you inwards away from outside distractions, whether these arise through sight, sound, or touch, and so on. Usually when we are not concentrated but fragmented our interest tends to wander off after everything that presents itself to our attention, but when we do Yoga we have to be attentive to our practice. We have to be present in what we are doing, to feel the touch of our feet on the floor, the vibration of the exhalation and the joy of stretching and lengthening the spine; this serves to concentrate our attention with the action of body and breath, to centre us as we withdraw from distractions.

For those who teach Yoga, it is easy to understand this redirection of the senses through the difference between practising Yoga yourself and teaching it to somebody else. When you practise you are introspective, attentive to the balance within yourself to the spine and to the breath; when you are teaching it is the opposite. You are wholly attentive to the student, looking and listening to what they are doing and to what they need.

Yoga is the stilling of the restless fluctuations of the mind so that the Eternal Self can be realized. Meditation is the means by which this may come about. The other steps of Yoga practice are a necessary foundation for this; in order to be wholly 'one pointed' (eka gratha) in your attention all your disparate elements have to become focused away from the ego and the transitory gratification of its desire for power and fulfilment, and surrendered to the Eternal Spirit within. So the practice of Patanjali's first five steps Yama, Niyama, Asana, Pranayama and Pratyahara slowly draw the different facets of your being, your daily life, your body, and your mind into harmony and you begin to discern the path more clearly through the fog of illusion, doubt, and dreams that obscure your vision at the beginning.

However the first five steps of Patanjali's Yoga system known as 'the outward path' cannot be accomplished without the practice of the inner path of the last three stages. The seeds of violence, untruthfulness, discontent and so on, lie in the subconscious as do the seeds of unsteadiness of posture and disquiet of breath. The practice of meditation, which helps eradicate these latencies, is a vital part of the whole eight faceted path. We cannot truly be practising Yoga by selecting one strand of its thread, although it is possible that those that attempt this can eventually be led to an awareness of its other aspects.

Meditation is not something that we 'do', it is rather a letting 'be'. It is allowing your thoughts, your preconceptions, your wish to succeed (however good your ambitions) and your anxieties to quieten and become silent. The gift of wholeness, holiness and love are within each of us, if only we can stop searching and 'doing' and be still and silent in body and thought, in the emotions and the deeper layers of the mind.

Dharana (Concentration)

We live in a state of continual distraction. Even when we are not actively engaged in 'thinking' about something we are day dreaming, fantasizing about the future, looking forward or fearful, reliving the past with longing, regret or guilt, worrying over trivia. When we sit and meditate we have to be attentive to the present moment, to be still and quiet in the only moment which is real, that is 'Now'. Memories and imagination are both distractions.

The difficulty is how to anchor our thoughts so that we have a hope of finding a moment of stillness and a place of silence amongst the shifting layers of the mind, even for an isolated second. This anchoring is Dharana. For Dharana we need a point of focus, a 'seed' from which the continuous concentration of the next step, Dhyana, can extend.

Meditation is a slow and therefore gentle process. Just as Asana should be a slow safe path to physical balance and stability, and Pranayama a gentle steadying of the psychic energy, so the mind has to find concentration step by step. We cannot sit and still our thoughts and contemplate the formless, timeless, eternal infinite without a point of focus. The shifting chattering mind cannot be stilled without an anchor to steady it down in concentration.

The journey of silence is difficult for most people, it can be boring, threatening, lonely. We can feel angry or humiliated when we discover how insecure and 'on the surface' we are.

Maybe we feel cheated because nothing happens, depressed because we are not getting anywhere. We have to let go the idea of achievement, particularly the achieving of religious experience. When for a split second the mind becomes still and a glimpse of truth is granted to us, as if a match was struck and lit for a moment the darkness of our perception, that moment is destroyed by our desire to catch and keep the experience. As we think 'how wonderful' and try to hold it we loose our anchor and the experience slides away into the past escaping our controlling ambition and its recapture becomes a fantasy of the future.

The practice of Yama and Niyama teach us that meditating in order to gain money or power is wrong but is less easy to let go of the wish for 'scriptural delights' (Patanjali, *Yoga Sutras*, Ch 1, v. 15).

The practice of meditation should make us less self-conscious and self-centred and less acquisitive of spiritual experience and reputation.

The mind, being prakrti (matter in Yoga philosophy), is subject to the three tendencies of Rajas, Tamas and Sattva. A mere cessation of restless activity does not necessarily bring clarity. We are more likely to sink into a Torpid Tamasic trance state that has nothing to do with Yoga. To become clear and 'one pointed' we need a focus for our attention to anchor it, fixing one thought in our minds to the exclusion of all other thoughts.

This focus of concentration can be in the form of sound (mantra), it can be visual (yantra), it can be felt through the breath. When you pay attention and concentrate your thought onto one point, this state usually alternates with the opposite tendency of your thoughts to drift, fragment and scatter. The goal of Yoga is to stop these fluctuating states of mind so that in total stillness you can be at one with the Spirit within you.

Dhyana (Meditation)

This is when concentration becomes continuous and unwavering, with the mind held to a single point where distractions cannot intrude. Just as there is a still point for the body that is the beginning and end of all movement, so with the mind there is a silence that is the beginning and end of all thought, where the creative Spirit of God has a chance of being revealed through the clamour of our distractions.

Samadhi (Illumination)

Union, Illumination, Enlightenment, call it what you will, is a completely different state of being, beyond the range of normal conscious awareness. Yoga draws together all the strands of human nature, body, mind and spirit so they are transformed and transcended and reality can be experienced. This is a resurrection of the body and mind where concentration is superfluous.

The practice of meditation

The search for transcendence, however, is not advanced by reading books but by practice: 'The fluctuations of the mind are restrained through practice, practice is the effort to secure steadiness.' (Patanjali, *Yoga Sutra*, Ch. 1). The practice of meditation is exceedingly simple. For most people this makes it exceedingly difficult. It is far easier to fascinate the mind with theories about what happens in meditation, or to bewitch the imagination with images of perfection, than it is to sit still and be silent. As with Asana practice you have to make a serious commitment to give time to meditation. Just as it takes time for your body to loosen up and let tension go, so it takes time to quieten down mentally particularly when you are beginning. Unless you have the discipline of a set length of time for meditation, you will give up and cut it short when you are distracted, or find an excuse to skip it altogether if you are 'not in the right mood'. This only exaggerates the tendency to be 'off centre' and scattered. In physical practice you can easily appreciate the need to spend time unwinding and letting go because you feel stiff and out of shape if you miss practising for too long. The mind, however, is more elusive than the body: you have to put aside a regular time on a daily basis. Just sitting down for a while when you happen to feel like a moment of peace and quiet may be therapeutic: it has nothing to do with meditation!

Practise meditation after Pranayama as this brings the body and mind to a quiet centred state. Decide how long you are going to sit: too short a time and you won't have a chance to become concentrated. Also decide on a maximum time: meditation is not 'having experiences' or 'enjoying a good meditation'; these can be just as distracting as worrying about what you are going to have for supper. A period of between 20 and 30 minutes is a good rule.

For most people it is fairly easy to find time for Pranayama and meditation early in the morning when the house is quiet; it is more difficult in the evening when you are distracted by the day's busy-ness. Twice daily practice makes an enormous difference; try to find time for a second period of meditation early in the evening if you can – if you leave it too late, when you are tired, concentration is harder and there is the added temptation to give up and leave it until tomorrow.

As with any other part of Yoga practice it is a question of finding the right balance for you – the balance between overambition and inertia. Between the Rajas and Tamas state so that there is a chance of Clarity.

Posture

The art of sitting and of silence is learned through both Asana and Pranayama. Any of the postures that are suitable for Pranayama can be used for meditation. You have to sit completely still: distractions arise in the body as well as in the mind. Ultimately bodily posture, breathing and mental concentration all come together. Meditation is not a matter of suppressing the physical; rather it is a bringing together of the body and mind to stillness and silence. In Yoga philosophy the body and the mind are both matter – Prakrti – the spirit within is Purusha.

Ways to meditate

There are as many ways to meditate as there are meditators; each of us has individual patterns of thought and tendencies to distraction. How you use the method of concentration you choose will, to some extent, depend on your background and conditioning. Not every method is going to suit everybody. Some people will concentrate easily on a sound, others on an image or breathing. Meditation is, above all, a matter of wholeness, of being within oneself in silence and stillness. It has nothing to do with fragmented dreams of imagination, ambition, memory or of ecstasy. It is the simple way of the narrow gate, the eye of the needle. It is also the beauty for which we have to be prepared to give up all we have, including our preconceived ideas of what meditation is. Therefore, whichever way we choose to meditate, it must be extremely simple and easily available to us from within the gift of our own experience. We can only start from where we are; any other beginning is false. We need therefore to use a method that comes from our own cultural or religious background, something with which we feel at home, an image or sound that can be our means of integration. Christians have, for example, used the name of Jesus as a form of meditation for centuries; it would be completely unsuitable for somebody from a different religious faith.

Mantra

This way of meditation uses a sacred word, sound or phrase as a focus of attention. It is practised widely at the present time and the *Hatha Yoga Pradipika* says, comfortingly, that it is suitable even for the most lax practitioner.

The prayer word or mantra is repeated silently from the beginning to the end of the meditation. The mantra is chosen carefully and is traditionally given by a Teacher to a disciple. It is a sacred word or phrase from the tradition to which the pupil belongs, but it is not a word that stimulates the imagination or sets up a train of discursive thought. Once given, the mantra is practised for life, the idea being that its vibrations become rooted in the subconscious and sound unceasingly. Mantras can be repeated in association with breathing or with the beat of the heart.

The supreme mantra is the sacred syllable AUM (OM), the eternal word, the word for God, the vibration of the creative force. Patanjali tells us to repeat this and to concentrate on its meaning. The mystic significance of Om is given in the *Mandukya Upanishad*.

The idea of repetitive sound affecting the mind is universal. Drumming and chanting have been used to affect our consciousness for thousands of years, and words have long been held to have magic power. Think of the difference between the shouting of an angry mob and the vibrations of a religious chant such as plainsong. Words, rhythms of breathing and sound are powerful tools. A mantra, therefore, should be given and accepted with care. It is a matter of great seriousness: mantras should not be doled out wholesale or sold like a franchise.

In Tantra and Hatha Yoga there are mantras associated with each of the chakras. The vibrations of these 'Bija' mantras are said to facilitate the raising of Kundalini (dormant energy, see page 11), for which purpose they would have to be repeated many hundreds of thousands of times.

Caution: Any practice based on ambition or the search for esoteric experience is a journey into the realms of the imagination and can therefore be a pathway to psychosis rather than to integration.

Visual meditation

We can also focus our attention through a visual image. This is a less popular method today than the use of sound as a mantra or a repetition of prayer (Japa). Perhaps this is because in the modern world we are assailed by images of one form or another, entertaining us or enticing us to buy and our visual sense is over stimulated so that the idea of concentration through that means is unappealing. Images have been objects of devotion in many different faiths, some being regarded as miraculous, and having the power to transmit knowledge of the divine.

The written symbol for the sacred sound OM, which can be sounded as a mantra, can be used for a visual meditation either on its own or incorporated in a pattern such as a Yantra or Mandala.

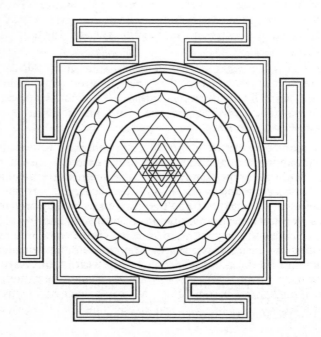

The Yantra is a geometric pattern that comes to and emerges from a central point. The shapes within the traditional pattern are symbolic of cosmic energies and powers associated with Tantra. In this practice, it is not just a question of 'looking at' the device as you might look at a religious picture or statue, but of concentrating on it and internalizing it. The Mandala in the Tibetan Buddhist tradition is used in the same way, it is a circular pattern with Gods and energies pictured within it.

Focus on the breath

In Classical Yoga focusing your attention on 'the inflowing and outflowing of the breath' is a recommended way of concentration. The breath is a natural mantra within us, given at birth and relinquished at death, more subtle than sound. The *Bhagavad Gita* speaks of breathing as being an act of renunciation whereby we 'offer the outflowing breath to the breath that flows in and the inflowing breath to the breath that flows out' (4 v 29). Through the note of the breath we can tune ourselves to the note of silence within us.

Distractions

Distractions come in various forms. As soon as you try to be silent all kind of chattering thoughts arise and it is with great difficulty that you are able to concentrate at all. 'Many branched and endless are the thoughts of the man who lacks determination' says the *Bhagavad Gita*, and you need determination and patience to continue to meditate as we all strike patches where the practice seems pointless as we are overwhelmed with seemingly irrelevant thoughts and doubts.

Patanjali classifies the distracting thoughts as Knowledge, Misconceptions, Imagination, Sleep and Memory. The most difficult of these is memory; memories are at the root of all of the other distractions and can lie deep in the subconscious, arising to disturb you at unexpected moments. This is particularly true when you have been practising Yoga and meditating for some time. As the mind begins to quieten it is as if the water of a lake becomes still and clear so that you begin to see things lying long submerged on the bottom. In the choppy weather of everyday living many things lie forgotten; when you change the pattern of your thoughts and become quiet they can emerge and demand your attention. In Yoga these old distractions from the past are called Samskaras and are thought to be the residue of more than one lifetime. Usually, although these Samskaras may only appear dimly in our dreams, they influence the way we react and make choices from day to day, which actions in their turn influence our future. The revelation and recognition of these tendencies brings the possibility of resolving and healing past hurts and conflicts so they no longer influence us. This is how Karma can be rendered inoperative through the practice of Yoga.

Obstacles

The problems which beset us in Yoga practice are listed in Patanjali's *Yoga Sutras* as Ignorance, Egoism, Attachment, Aversion and the Fear of Death. Ignorance (Avidya) literally translated as 'not seeing' is the root cause of the others, confusing the Ego with the Spirit of God within us and so clouding our motives for Yoga practice. Self-interest can never be the foundation of morality or of any religious discipline such as Yoga, which must be based on self-surrender and detachment: 'Set thy heart upon thy work but never on its reward' (*Bhagavad Gita*, 4 v 47).

Powers

As the Asanas change your body, and its use of physical energy becomes more economical, so too the practice of mental concentration, which sweeps away some of the extraneous mental clutter, allows us to function more effectively. Many people who meditate find that the patterns of their life change as they become less distracted in general. You may notice the world around you in a different way, enjoy deeper personal relationships, be less antagonistic in responding to annoying circumstances, want less background noise and distraction in your life. When you do watch television or listen to music you may enjoy it more. Times of silence and stillness are bound to affect our lives; it is these conditions, rather than 'experiences' or 'ecstasies' which are very often merely ego-based distractions, that are the real fruits of meditation. As our energy changes and rebalances at a physical level, so it changes at a psychic level too. The Siddis (supernormal powers) mentioned in Patanjali's third chapter, are talents that we all possess in some degree or another, although they are usually dormant. These include telepathy, healing, clairvoyance, seeing auras, and so on. Just as some people are born with more developed talents for music or art, there are some born with psychic abilities – abilities which it is also possible to induce through drugs, just as abnormal physical development can be induced (Patanjali, *Yoga Sutras,* 4 v 1). Very occasionally, as the psychic energy changes, these Siddhis manifest themselves for a short while before disappearing as balance is re-established. They are phenomena on the psychic level and have no spiritual significance whatsoever. They can be an obstacle to the practice of Yoga as your ego becomes fascinated with them and inflated and self-important, and you can be caught in the trap that waits at every turn of Yoga practice. The temptation of trying to achieve and hold on to what you can do, whether it is a question of struggling to 'do' the Asanas or of meditating in order to 'be' special.

'Day after day let the Yogi practise harmony of soul: in a secret place, in deep solitude, master of his mind, hoping for nothing, desiring nothing.' (*Bhagavad Gita,* 6 v 10).

'free from attachment to sensory pleasures and also ideas of Spiritual attainment'. (Patanjali, *Yoga Sutras,* Ch. 1).

Meditation practice guidelines

1 Set aside 20 to 30 minutes morning and evening and stick to it.
2 Practise Pranayama before you sit to meditate.
3 Sit still straight and relaxed.
4 Adopt one method of concentration and stay with that from beginning to the end each day, every day for the full time of your meditation.
5 When you find you have become distracted, gently return to your meditation.
6 A guide or a friend who is already meditating is beyond price; there are more people in this category than you might think, but they may be difficult to recognize. Take your time and if you have a problem you will find the person who is right for you.

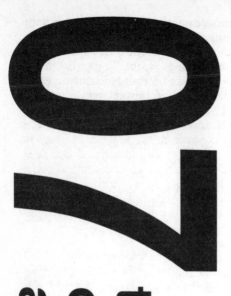

07

therapeutic use of Yoga Asanas and Pranayama

In this chapter you will learn:
- how to use Yoga to overcome physical problems
- how to cope with stress
- how to release tension to encourage healing.

Sickness is one of the 'distractions of the mind' mentioned in the *Yoga Sutras* as being an impediment to practice. Asanas and Pranayama help to counteract this, but they do very much more, working against other distractions from Yoga, listed by Patanjali, which have a less obvious physical correction: inertia, doubt, delusion, laziness, intemperance, mistaken ideas and the inability to concentrate and to remain concentrated.

Many people start Yoga at a time of crisis, when they feel impelled to do something to help themselves, something to change the pattern of their lives and when they are prepared to give time for this. Maybe it is a physical crisis or an emotional trauma, or they realize that life is becoming stressful and they want to reverse the process. Because of this Yoga is sometimes thought of as a kind of therapy and it can be used as such, though it is of course, very much more.

Physical health is a by-product of Yoga practice, which embraces the whole human being from skin to soul. As Yoga postures and breathing are intended to balance the structure and functioning of the body, they will always have a therapeutic effect, and Yoga practice is one of the best preventive health regimes you could possibly undertake.

You have the most incredible healing powers within yourself which are largely unrealized and unused – powers of the mind and of the body. When you are sick, the intelligent use of postures and breathing can help you cure yourself by allowing the natural healing abilities you already possess a better chance of working. They are an aid to the unconscious rebalancing and regeneration that goes on in the body from the day you are born.

Usually healing is a slow and gentle process, although you may have to work hard to focus your attention to undo long-standing muscular distortions and restricted joints. Very, very occasionally breathing and postures can have a sudden dramatic result, but this is the exception and not the rule, and even if this occurs you need to go on practising to keep the old patterns which helped cause the problem, from re-establishing themselves.

If you decide to use Yoga postures to help yourself, don't practise another discipline that might conflict with its aims, for example, there is no point doing Yoga postures for osteo-arthritis and also lifting weights and doing aerobics.

Important guidelines

1 Always consult a qualified doctor. Be sensible – asking advice of a doctor means that you will get a qualified opinion without which you might make a disastrous mistake.
2 Use your common sense and listen to your body – many exotic claims have been made for Yoga over the centuries. Anything that is going to work has its roots in the physical body, there is no point in thinking only in terms of prana and chakras when the obvious problem is a crooked spine or bad breathing pattern.
3 Keep it simple by sticking to a regular daily routine.

Yoga Asanas for spinal problems and backache

Distorted posture stresses the physical structure. Body weight is shifted out of line, muscles have to tighten unnecessarily and this can have far-reaching effects – in your breathing, circulation, digestion, and so on. Bad posture may not always result in backache, but it will always cause stress somewhere in the body and should always be corrected.

First, lie in the recuperation pose (page 76). Exhale and let your spine lengthen and relax. If it is difficult to lie flat, use cushions under your head and/or put your legs on a chair so that the backs of your calves are supported. Raise your arms up in the air and with an outbreath cross them and let them drop down across your chest. Lying with the arms crossed like this means that the shoulder blades move outwards away from the spine; you can then feel the whole of your back from the base of your neck to the back of your hips in contact with the floor. Stay in this position for at least ten minutes releasing tension as you exhale and letting the back of your body relax down into the ground.

All the standing positions except the triangle pose, can be practised. Take care not to go too far at first and be sure to keep in line, lengthening from your hips to your head. For the standing forward bends, use a chair or table to keep your hips and your head in line as you lengthen forwards (see page 29).

After a few weeks try a modified shoulderstand. Lie on your back in the recuperation pose; your feet should be near your hips and parallel. Be sure that you are lying straight with the back of your neck long and relaxed and your chin in line with the notch between your collar bones. As you breathe out and your abdominal muscles contract let the back of your waist touch the floor and curling your spine let your tail bone and then your hips lift off the floor. As you lift up the back of your body should lengthen from the back of your head towards your feet, which stay down with the weight on your heels. As you come down let your spine roll gently back onto the ground. This is the bridge pose (Setubandhasana). After a few weeks do the same movement with your feet raised on the seat of a chair (be sure the chair can't slip). When you can lift your hips up further you can put your hands on your back ribs. Then try rolling up into a proper shoulderstand (see page 39) and observe the cautions.

To release the upper spine lie prone and do the locust pose on page 64.

Also do the supine twist on page 48.

See also the section on hips.

Feet

Few people in the West have really good feet, and while they may not notice that they work less than perfectly when we are young, they become an increasing problem when we get older. Our feet, composed of many small bones, should be strong supple and springy, acting as shock absorbers. How they function affects our knees and our hips and, through these the way the lower spine balances between the hip bones. The flexibility of the soles of the feet, together with the action of the legs, helps the venous blood return to the heart thus preventing varicose veins. Toes that spread and adjust help us maintain our balance. In their natural state feet do not taper towards a point but are square across the ends of the toes. It is extremely rare to find shoes that allow for this.

To straighten and strengthen the feet and toes

1 Sit on the heels as on page 51 with the heels touching each other. Loop a belt round the ankles if they come apart. If this is painful because the feet are stiff, try putting a rolled towel under them and/or putting a cushion over your heels.

2 Sit on your heels with your toes tucked under so that the soles of the feet stretch. Stay in this position for a minute or two. If your feet are stiff go very slowly, a little bit at a time.

3 Stand straight as on page 25 with your weight on your heels and the outsides of your feet, keeping the big toes on the floor. Lift the inner arches of your feet up and pressing the balls of your feet down, lift up all of your toes. Repeat several times.

4 Stand straight with the weight on your heels, and toes spread out touching the ground. Lift up your big toe keeping the others on the floor. If this is not possible, hold the other four toes down while you lift the big toe up. Soon you will be able to move it independently.

5 Then, spreading out all your toes, keep the little toe and the big toe on the ground and lift up the middle three. If you can't do this, hold the little and big toes down and lift the middle three up. This way you can re-educate your muscles so that the transverse arch of the foot becomes strong.

A bunion is the bump that forms at the base of the big toe when it has been pushed over towards the other toes, instead of being in a straight line with the inside edge of the foot. Even at a late stage, a lot can be done to correct this. Walk with bare feet whenever possible. Nearly all shoes taper towards a point (even if only slightly, as in the case of men's shoes) whereas feet are square across the toes. You have to be extremely fussy about shoes if you want to walk beautifully into old age. If the big toes have deviated practise standing straight with a short strap (your watch strap would do) looped across between your big toes so that they are pulled towards each other and straightened. This will give you the feeling of what it is like to stand with the feet working properly. Most people have completely lost any concept of this. You can also loop the strap between your big toes in shoulderstand when the feet are not bearing any weight. Pull you heels slightly apart so that the toes are stretched out towards each other.

Knees

The knee is basically a hinge that bends and straightens with just a small amount of rotation. The hip is a ball and socket joint which has a large range of movement. In Yoga practice many people hurt their knees trying to force movements in the knee when the thighs are in fact restricted by lack of movement in the hip. For example, the lotus position requires a lot of outward rotation in the hips and not an extraordinary movement in the knees. You can injure your knees by trying to force the legs into this position when the hips are stiff. Long-standing knee problems are usually accompanied by an uneven movement in the hips, or a badly aligned foot, or both.

Postures for knees

1 Practise standing straight (page 25) with the feet parallel and the weight on your heels and the outsides of the feet with the big toes down on the ground. (The centre line of the feet should be parallel – that is, the line from the centre of the heel to the point between the base of the second and third toe.) Your knees should face straight ahead with the feet, and the inner arches of the feet should lift up. If standing like this is hard you may need to do the exercises for feet above. Feel how the footprints touch the floor; they should, of course, be even. Stretch your knees straight.

2 Sit in the wide legged sitting position (page 50). If this is difficult because the muscles at the back of the legs are tight, sit against a wall. The backs of your legs must be as flat on the floor as possible. Exhale and let the backs of your legs feel heavy and the hollows behind the knees open and go down to touch the ground.

3 Hyperextended knees – In some people the backs of the knees are overstretched, so that the leg bows backwards at the top of the calf. In this case, keeping the weight on your heels in the standing poses, be sure that the knees are not 'snapped back' with pressure behind the knee; this may feel as if your legs are not quite straight. When doing the standing forward bends be sure that your hips stay directly above your heels.

Hips

Many people in Western societies have a limited range of movement in the hips because they seldom sit on the floor or squat, and lie in cots or push-chairs as babies instead of being carried across their mother's backs. Poor movement in the hips can throw extra strain on the lower back, and many people with lower back problems need to work at loosening up their hips.

Postures for hips

1 Bound angle pose (page 53). Sit leaning against a wall with the soles of the feet together and cushions underneath each thigh. Exhale and let your legs go down onto the cushions. Keep your lower back in contact with the wall. Stay exhaling and dropping the thighs with each breath for some minutes – stiff hips need time. After a few breaths, when you are able to let go in the hips, you can take away the cushions. (You need the cushions to start with, otherwise it feels as if you are going to stretch too suddenly in the groins, and this inhibits you from releasing the stiffness). The half bound angle pose (page 54) can also be practised like this with your back against a wall and a cushion under the bent knee.

2 Hero's pose (page 52) can be done sitting on one or several books. Gradually reduce the height until you are sitting on the floor; this may take some months of regular practice.

3 All the standing poses particularly tree pose 1 and 2 (pages 26 and 28).

4 The supine leg stretches (page 47) using a belt looped round the foot.

5 Inverted poses which take the weight off the legs can be helpful in moving a stiff or arthritic joint. If you can do headstand or shoulderstand, stay in the position for some minutes lengthening upwards with the elbows well planted on the floor. As you exhale keep the legs very straight so that they go up away from the hips, then do the one leg down positions (page 42). You can also take the leg down to the side. If you cannot do either of the inverted poses straight enough or for long enough to practise these one-legged stretches, then do shoulderstand and when you have rolled down do the supine leg stretches while still lying on your back.

6 Cow pose (page 61). Do the hip movement only.

Caution: These poses should work on the hip joints and not pull on the knees. If you feel any pain in the knees you have gone too far.

Arthritis in the hip is an extremely painful condition. People with arthritis tend to breathe in a shallow frightened way when they approach a movement which they expect to hurt. Instead, try breathing slowly, gently and deeply as you move, letting the exhaling breath dissolve the barriers which can be partly fear and tension. Holding the breath and pushing into the pain as if pushing into a brick wall will get you nowhere.

Shoulders

Nearly everyone has one shoulder stiffer than the other because of being right- or left-handed. With modern technology we use our full range of movement less and small restricted movements more, pushing buttons, telephoning, using computers. All these tense the shoulders without giving the arms a chance to stretch out fully and release. Combined with the tension in the shoulders that comes from anxiety and emotional distress this can cause a lot of problems and tight stiff shoulders are extremely common. Tight shoulders can also help pull the head out of line and contribute to headaches.

Postures for shoulders

1 Cow pose (page 61). With the arms only, while standing straight. Keep your weight on your heels and the back of your waist long. If you can't touch your hands together, catch each end of a belt. Never force or grapple your hands together – breathe out and release tension then the shoulders will free themselves.

2 Eagle pose (page 28). With the arms only. If this is difficult at the beginning, just hug your arms across your chest and later, when the back of your shoulders have released, cross the wrists.

3 Salute position 1 (page 69). With the hands up your back palms together and fingers pointing upwards as on page 29. If this is hard at first, just hold your elbows behind your back. Be sure to keep the back of your waist long and do not stick your chest out.

4 All the standing poses (pages 25–33) are good for shoulders.

5 Dog pose (page 34).

Eyes

Modern technology also focuses strain and tension in the eyes. Even before the invention of television and computer screens, there was a steadily increasing dependence on our visual sense. There are more instructions to read, more advertisements to see and more written signs to be followed than ever before. For this reason alone some kind of relaxation should be practised for the eyes, even if no other Yoga exercise is done at all. If eye strain is a problem and you wish to meditate it is better not to focus on a visual image.

1 To relax the eyes, Sanmukhi Mudra is helpful. This is explained in the Pranayama chapter (page 79).
2 Trataka helps to train the eye muscles. It involves gazing at a fixed point or series of points. This is not as simple as it sounds, as at first you tend to try staring too hard and tensing the back of the neck. Rather than try this on your own it would be better to seek a qualified instructor.
3 Cooling breath (Sitali) and alternate nostril breathing from the Pranayama chapter are helpful with eye problems.

Caution: The eyes are delicate organs which are placed in the protective bony box of the skull at the top of the spine for very good reasons. If you are suffering from eye problems connected with diabetes or have a feeling of pressure in the eyes when practising do not do any of the inverted poses without seeking medical advice, and be careful with positions where the head is lowered such as Salute to the Sun (page 69), or the front and back bends where this occurs.

Stress

Stress manifests itself in many different ways and is thought to be a contributory factor to a large variety of different ailments. You can be stressed by your work (or lack of it), your environment, by your partner (or lack of one), by bereavement, by emotional trauma; the list seems endless. You can even be stressed by overtraining your body in order to keep fit. Yoga, which is a whole way of life that entails listening to yourself, being sensitive to your body's real needs and treating it with love and respect, is the perfect antidote to stress.

Postures and breathing for stress

This programme can be done at any time. If you are feeling particularly stressed you can do it twice a day, followed in the morning by the Yoga postures that you usually practise. If you are beginning Yoga and you are under stress, practise this programme twice a day (morning and evening) for a month and then follow the morning session with the beginner's programme (page 103). When things improve then do the normal Yoga positions in the morning. Continue to do the stress programme in the evening as long as you consider it helpful.

1 Lie on you back in the recuperation pose (page 76). Your spine should lie long and flat on the floor and your feet should be close to your hips with the knees pointing towards the ceiling. If your head does not rest comfortably on the floor with the neck long and relaxed, place a folded towel under your head. If your back is arched, then rest the backs of your legs on a chair. As you exhale, let your abdomen go in and the back of your waist drop down onto the ground so that your spine is completely resting on the floor. As the breath comes in leave the back of your body in contact with the floor. Stay like this, breathing slowly and gently for at least five minutes.

2 Then fold your legs towards your trunk wrapping your arms round your thighs. Don't tighten your shoulders but just let the weight of your arms hug your knees towards your trunk. Stay for one or two minutes.

3 Child pose (page 51). Sit on your heels as on page 50 (if necessary put a rolled towel under your feet and/or a cushion over your heels). Bend forwards and rest your arms and head on a cushion placed on the floor in front of you. If you are stiff you can do this forward stretch sitting on a chair with your arms and head resting on a table in front of you. Bend your arms and hold your elbows resting your head on them. Whichever position you are in, drop your hips down, let your back ribs expand as you breathe in, and feel your back grow longer as you breathe out, relaxing your neck and shoulders

4 Then sit up and keeping your hips down exhale and turn to the left as your back lengthens and your abdomen goes in.

Keep your shoulders relaxed. The movement is from the spine which stays centred and grows tall. Stay for two or three breaths and then come back to the centre and do the position on the other side.

5 Stand straight and do the arm positions given in the section for stiff shoulders (page 125).

6 Now you can either continue with the rest of your usual practice or do triangle pose and one other standing pose followed by shoulderstand (page 39).

7 Follow this by the supine twist (page 48).

8 Then do corpse pose (page 77).

For Pranayama you can do simple deep breathing (page 90) or interval breathing on the exhalation (page 91).

Diet

In Yoga diet is based on the balance of the three tendencies Tamas (inertia), Rajas (activity) and Sattva (clarity) (see page 6). Here you have to use your common sense as needs vary widely, dictated by climate, age and physical type as well as work done and the state of your health. Someone living today in a cold climate will need a different type of diet from that prescribed in India 1000 years ago in an ancient Yoga text.

The following categories are a rough guide:

- **Rajas food:** Hot spicy seasonongs, tea, coffee, salt, unripe food, egg, meat and fish.
- **Tamas food:** Stale food, over-ripe fruit, alcohol, fermented food or drink, root vegetables, fried food.
- **Sattvic food:** Fruit, vegetables except as above, cereals, milk, honey, seeds, nuts, pulses and butter.

How food is treated also affects its tendency; overcooking food makes it more Tamasic, for example. So eat food that is grown and treated as naturally as possible with a large proportion of raw or short cooked food. If you try to stay as near to the Sattvic list as you can you will eat very well, but our present day knowledge of minerals and vitamins needs to be taken into account. The other aspects of Yoga that need to be thought about are Tapas (austerity), which would exclude over indulgence, Saucha (purity), which would indicate food as uncontaminated as possible and Yama (non-violence) (See Patanjali's eight limbs page 6).

Therapy

Addiction

The discipline of Yoga practice can help break compulsive patterns of behaviour, but only if it is part of a serious programme of total abstinence combined with medical help and counselling. Do standing Asanas and, if flexible, Salute to the Sun (page 69) and shoulderstand. Relaxation and interval breathing and also alternate nostril breathing (page 94) are helpful. This is one of the instances where it is better to use a breathing technique than to do simple deep breathing.

Anxiety

Shoulder stretches (page 125) and shoulderstand (page 39), Kapalabhati (page 81), Viloma on the exhalation (page 91), lion breath (page 96).

Arthritis

See pages 120–25 for the poses for structural problems. Start your practice with the recuperation pose (page 76) and spend at least five minutes breathing slowly and deeply in this position before doing the other postures. Practise the interval breathing on the exhalation (page 91). Do not attempt the inverted poses if there is arthritis in the neck.

Asthma

Do all the standing poses and all the poses in the section on shoulders (page 125). Practise Kapalabhati (page 81), interval breathing on the exhalation (page 91) and the Recuperation Pose with abdominal breathing as above.

Colitis

Practise the stress programme.

Constipation

Sun salute (page 69) and shoulderstand and as many of the shoulderstand and plough variations as you are able to do. Deep breathing and a long relaxation.

Depression

Standing poses, Salute to the Sun, vibration breathing and lion breath.

Diabetes

Any of the Yoga poses are good but be careful with the inverted poses as sometimes there is a complication with eye problems, so ask your doctor about this. Practise Kapalabhati and vibration breathing.

Disc problems

See the section on the spine (page 120). When the condition is acute do relaxation with deep breathing in the recuperation pose only. Avoid all forward bending movements with the legs straight until the condition has improved.

Epilepsy

Cases are so different that you have to experiment a bit. Active exercise followed immediately by relaxation has been known to trigger fits so go slowly and sit quietly in a meditation pose rather than doing corpse pose at the end of your practice. You can relax at another time. Shoulderstand (page 39) is good, as are all the poses in the shoulder section (page 125). Avoid Kapalabhati, vibration breathing and holding your breath.

Headache

Relax in corpse pose with a small pad (a tightly folded sock) in between your shoulder blades under your spine. Then practise the supine twist. Regular practise of shoulderstand helps with migraine but don't try it when you have a headache. Do deep breathing and interval breathing. Relax with a rice bag over your eyes (page 86).

Hypertension

Follow the stress routine, avoid inverted poses and salute to the sun when the blood pressure is raised. Do standing forward bends going forward to a chair. Do the shoulder poses (page 125), standing poses and sitting poses. Ujayii breathing and Viloma on the exhalation.

Insomnia

Practise shoulderstand, plough (feet on a chair), supine leg stretches and supine twist before you go to bed. If you wake up in the night do the supine twist, Kapalabhati and then deep breathing.

Multiple sclerosis

You need to keep mobile without getting fatigued and for this Yoga is ideal. Ability varies so much there are few set rules, except that regular practice is essential, little and often and always do a good relaxation at the end. It is possible to adapt the poses so that many of them can be done from a chair; the forward bends, shoulder movements and twists for example. A qualified teacher should be able to help you with this. Practise vibration breathing.

Osteoporosis

You need to keep active and mobile so Yoga Asanas are fine. There is more need than ever to keep the spine long so that there is no compression of the vertebrae. Take great care with twists and inverted poses. Weight bearing exercises are beneficial, so practise standing poses, salute to the sun, hand balances.

Piles

The inverted poses can help, also backbends lying prone on the floor (page 64).

Pregnancy

Yoga practice can be continued throughout pregnancy although some of the poses will have to be adapted to accommodate the growing baby. Any movement that contracts the abdomen such as sitting twists and extreme front bends must be avoided, as should Kapalabhati. Find a qualified teacher to advise you. Failing this there are specialized books on the subject. Also see page 134.

Varicose veins

The inverted poses and as many of the variations of shoulderstand as you can do. Check with your doctor first.

Many people start to practise Yoga because they have an aching back or are suffering from stress-related problems, and in the course of relieving these learn to face reality and be gentle with themselves as they discover the strains and tensions that have to be worked through. This can be a true understanding of the Yoga principle of 'non-violence' and the need to live in a more balanced way, which can have far-reaching effects on the individual and on society.

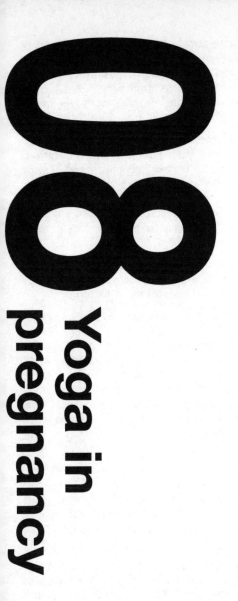

08

Yoga in pregnancy

In this chapter you will learn:
- to adapt Yoga postures during pregnancy
- how Yoga teaching is changing in today's Western world.

Yoga during pregnancy is extremely fashionable at the moment with many books and teachers recommending women take up Yoga as a form of antenatal exercise and preparation for birth. This has not always been the case, as until very recently there were teachers who were against the practice of Yoga during pregnancy.

For women who are already practising Yoga regularly and who have a good understanding of their strengths and limitations Yoga can indeed be a wonderful way of keeping fit and healthy during pregnancy and of preparing for labour and delivery. Pregnancy is a time when most women have an increased sense of body awareness and their understanding of Yoga can be enormously enhanced by continuing to practise during these months.

Pregnancy, labour and motherhood are all hard work and women need strength, stamina and energy as well as flexibility to be able to enjoy this time and to fulfil their potential.

The physical changes of pregnancy can tax women's strength and put strains on the structure of the body so this is when posture and strong muscles are more important than ever. For example the weight of the growing baby can pull you forwards, increasing the curve at the back of your waist causing backache as the muscles of the lower back contract to pull the upper body back in line with gravity and re-establish postural balance. The practice of standing poses during these months keeps your posture well balanced, your joints supple and exercises your back muscles.

This is certainly not a time to stop practising but you will have to adapt your usual programme to accommodate the needs of your growing child, for example bending forwards with your legs together will soon become impossible so you will have to have more space between your legs to make room for the baby as you fold forwards.

When twisting the more advanced poses will put too much pressure on your abdomen in the later stages of pregnancy as will the poses where you lie prone. This will rule out the full version of the Salute to the Sun but the short version can still be practised with the Child pose in the middle of the sequence slightly adapted. Whether you continue to practise the inverted poses in later pregnancy is a matter of choice. Some women who are already practising them regularly continue to do so all the way through, finding them a relief from the heaviness and stiffness of the last few weeks before the birth. Most women however prefer not to practise these poses in the last two or three months.

Above all this is a time for common sense and listening to your body, being sensitive to the changes taking place. If you are in any doubt you should seek qualified medical advice.

Relaxation and breathing are the aspects of Yoga that are of vital importance during labour. The poses give you the advantage of mobility and strength, which can be of enormous value when giving birth, but the ability to relax for a few minutes between contractions during a long labour and knowing how to focus on your breathing and to control it without panic will increase your stamina and endurance beyond measure.

Yoga practice is not going to guarantee a short pain-free labour and an easy delivery but however the birth of your baby happens to be you will be better prepared through your practice and experience.

Whether the delivery is easy or difficult you will find that you have a huge advantage as women who do Yoga recover quickly from childbirth and you can start a gentle recovery programme almost straight away with straight stretches either lying down or standing, and shoulder stretches that release your upper back. Nursing a baby can make you round shouldered so be sure to have a counter-stretch.

Whether there is an advantage in taking up Yoga as a form of antenatal exercise when you have never practised it before is more doubtful. Yoga is a profound practice and the poses and breathing can have far reaching effects, which should be taken seriously. Many women enrol in special classes based on Yoga, which are specifically for expectant mothers, and have found something of value, which has encouraged them later in life to enrol in a class and start practising seriously. But most new mothers are very unlikely to have the time to establish a regular routine of practice with just a few months' previous experience, nor should they. At this time their priorities should be for their new baby and family and they do not need to be burdened with a feeling of inadequacy because they have not the time for a practice that they have not had the opportunity to fully understand.

If you should want to start Yoga during your pregnancy, you would need to find a very experienced teacher giving private lessons or lessons in a small group, and you would need to plan to give time for this. A good antenatal class might prove more valuable. There is no harm in waiting a little longer to do Yoga until your baby needs you a little less of the time.

Asanas that should NOT be practised during pregnancy

- Dog pose with head up (page 35)
- Inverted Lotus poses (pages 44 and 45)
- Sage's twists (pages 62 and 63)
- Locust pose (page 64)
- Upwards Bow pose (page 65)
- Tortoise pose (page 57)
- Salute to the Sun (page 69)
- Plough pose with the knees to the ears (page 46)
- Fish pose (page 60)
- Any other pose where you feel that you are constricting your growing baby.

Asanas that have to be adapted during late pregnancy

- Standing forward bends (page 32). Make more space between your legs as you go forwards so as not to press on your abdomen.
- Supine twist (page 48). Your legs will not be able to fold in so tightly.
- Sitting forward bends (page 49). Keep your legs slightly apart and don't go too far down.
- Sitting forward bends (pages 54–57) Don't go too far down.
- Salute to the Sun, shorter version (page 76). Fold into Child pose (page 51) with the legs slightly apart.
- Plough pose (page 40). Raise your legs onto the seat of a chair.

Pranayama that should NOT be practised during pregnancy

- Kapalabhati (page 81)
- Kumbaka (page 92). Practise Viloma instead to control breathing without panic.
- Lion Breath (page 96)

Yoga today

In the middle of the last century few people living in the affluent Western world had heard of Yoga. Today it is a widely publicised, fashionable form of exercise practised by pop stars and movie actors as well as many thousands of ordinary men and women worldwide.

Yoga Asanas and Pranayama have certainly come a long way following the Second World War when the interest in Eastern religion and spirituality blossomed. The courageous and inspired teachers who travelled to the West have had their efforts well rewarded. Yoga has ceased to be the interest of a small minority and has become mainstream.

This has had many advantages but there are also some drawbacks.

Yoga has gained popularity along with the cult of fitness, the gym and the body beautiful. Long gone are the days when the world famous teacher B. K. S. Iyengar could write in his best selling book *Light on Yoga* that all you need for the practice of Asanas is a clean airy place, a blanket and determination. Today's would be students are likely to find Yoga taught in specially designed centres equipped with various aids to practice such as belts, blocks and back-stretchers, as well as mats and mirrors. The commercial pressures of setting up and maintaining such places mean that the way Yoga is taught has had to change. Forms of Yoga where a single instructor can teach large numbers have become the norm, with regular attendance at a class being encouraged. For many people Yoga is considered to be a group activity with grades of classes through which one can progress. Famous visiting instructors give special courses and Yoga holidays in peaceful venues are on offer. Yoga may or may not bring you the benefits of health, fitness, tranquility, enlightenment, sexual prowess etc. promised in the publicity but it can certainly make you poorer financially.

The marketing of Yoga also means that there needs to be a brand name to sell and nowadays it is considered normal for the ancient sacred word 'Yoga' to be prefixed by the name of the teacher who has put his trademark on the particular form of practice being taught. In fact most would-be students demand to know which brand you are selling when they enquire about classes. As each teacher will to some extent interpret what they have learnt in their own way it may be more sensible to make your choice by considering the individual rather than the brand name they are teaching.

The fastest growing Yoga in the popularity stakes at the moment is Ashtanga Yoga as taught in Mysore in India and also worldwide by J. P. S. Pattabhi Jois. This is the practice that is closest to the Western gymnastic, aerobic workout and many people take it up as an alternative. Yoga has been taught in many places in India besides the traditional ashrams, and fast jumping sequences similar to Astanga Yoga have been taught in schools and colleges to young people for many years. Whether older people whose bodies tend to be stiffer and more set in habitual patterns of movement can benefit in the long term from practising these sequences in a large group with little correction is open to doubt. But many find the practice more enjoyable than the visit to the gym and come to an understanding of Yoga through this introduction.

Among the many other notable teachers who have had an important influence in the West is B. K. S. Iyengar, who originally travelled to the West to teach the famous Indian thinker Krishnamurti.

Iyengar Yoga is one of the most widely practised forms of Yoga and there are Iyengar Institutes worldwide.

Both B. K. S. Iyengar and Patthabi Jois were at one time pupils of the legendary Tirumali Krishnamacharya, whose son T. V. K. Desikachar has written a moving account of his father's life and teaching. Sri Desikachar, who also numbered Krishnamurti amongst his students still teaches in his father's home town of Chennai (Madras) and also travels worldwide. In his lifetime Krishnamacharya refused to allow anyone to call him guru or even a Yogi.

taking it further

Classic texts

The Upanishads, translated by Juan Mascaro, Penguin
The Bhagavad Gita, translated byJuan Mascaro, Penguin
A Source Book in Indian Philosophy, Radhakrishnan and
   Moore, Princetown
RajaYoga, Vivekananda, Ramakrishna Vedanta Centre
Yoga Philosophy of Patanjali, Swami Hariharananda Aranya,
   Calcutta University

Contemporary books

Light on Yoga, B. K. S. Iyengar, Thorsons
A best-selling book by a world renowned Guru. More than
600 photographs of the author performing Yoga Asanas from
simple to very advanced positions.

Yoga Mala, J. P. S. Pattabhi Jois, Productions 2000
The author is the founder of the popular Ashtanga Yoga
movement.

Yoga, Mind and Body, Sivananda Yoga Vedanta Centre,
Dorling Kindersley
An attractively produced book aimed at the Western market.
It is based on the teaching of Sri Swami Sivananda and Swami
Vishnu Devananda. Colour photography and an easily
understood text. The Sivananda network has teachers in
many countries.

Health, Healing and Beyond, Yoga and the Living Tradition of Krishnamacharya, T. V. K. Desikachar, Aperture

This is the author's tribute to his father and is an inspiring story of a man whose students have taught Yoga all over the world. One hundred years old when he died, the late Krishnamacharya seems to have had a commonsense and independent approach as well as being a devoted practitioner of a traditional, commonsense and independent approach as well as being a devoted practitioner of traditional Yoga.

Yoga, the Spirit and Practice of Moving into Stillness, Erich Shiffman, Pocket Books

Yoga from a Western point of view. The author travelled extensively to learn Yoga. He now teaches the stars in his home state of California.

Karma Kola, Geeta Mehta, Vintage

An Indian perspective of "the marketing of the mystic east". Very funny but also very sad.

Madame Blatvatsky's Baboon, Peter Washington, Schocken

This book is about "the rise of the Western Guru" and is an interesting account of some of the movements and cults associated with the increased interest in Eastern Spirituality in the last century. A good antidote to some of the more beguiling groups around today.

Spirit of Yoga, Kathy Phillips, Cassell

There is a lot of fun to be got out of reading this overview of the present day Yoga scene and some of its crazier manifestations, but the author has practised Yoga for more than 20 years so there is also a serious side to this book. A down to earth account of Yoga practice with beautiful illustrations.

The Yoga Tradition of the Mysore Palace, N. E. Sjoman, Abhinav Publications

The late Maharaja of Mysore was a Yoga enthusiast. This book is the result of the author's research in the archives of the palace. There are pictures of the postures taken from some of the old texts.

Websites

British Wheel of Yoga is recognised by the Sports Council as the governing body for Yoga in Great Britain – http://shrewsbury.dsvr.co.uk/~bwy/

Ashtanga Yoga – http:///ashtanga.org/index.shmtl

Iyengar Yoga – http://www.bksiyengar.com/topband.htm

Sivananda Yoga – http://www.sivananda.org/

The Spirit and Practice of Moving into Stillness with Erich Shiffman – http://www.movingintostillness.com/index.htm

glossary

Ahimsa   Non-violence, one of Patanjali's Yamas.

Anga   Limb. There are eight angas in Patanjali's Yoga system.

Apana   Vital air – constitute of Prana.

Aparigraha   Not hoarding, one of Patanjali's Yamas.

Asana   Posture. The third of Patanjali's eight limbs.

Asteya   Not stealing, one of Patanjali's Yamas.

Atman   Immortal soul.

AUM or OM   The Sanskrit syllable or sound for the Absolute.

Avidya   Ignorance. The principle impediment to Yoga.

Bandha   A lock.

Bakhti Yoga   The path of adoration or devotion.

Bramacharya   Continence. One of Patanjali's Yamas.

Buddha   Enlightened One. The founder of the Buddhist faith, formerly Gautama.

Buddhi   Intellect.

Chakra   Wheel – energy centre in the subtle body.

Dharana   Concentration. The sixth of Patanjali's eight limbs.

Dhyana   Meditation. The seventh of Patanjali's limbs.

Eka Gratha   One-pointed.

Gautama   Another name for Buddha, the Enlightened One.

Guna   Quality or tendency. The shifting balance of the three Gunas, Rajas, Tamas, and Sattva cause the creation of the Cosmos in Yoga philosophy.

Guru   Teacher. Literally 'one who brings light'.

Hatha Yoga   Yoga through physical discipline.

Ida   The nadi (pathway) in the subtle body that carries the lunar energy.

Isvara Pranidhana   Devotion to God. One of Patanjali's Niyamas.

Japa   Repetition as a means of prayer.

Jnana Yoga   Yoga through discriminative knowledge.

Kapalabhati   A cleansing breathing process, a kriya.

Karma   Action. The rule by which actions have an effect on the future.

Karma Yoga   Yoga through selfless action.

Kosha   Envelope or sheath of subtle energy.

Kriya   Cleansing process.

Kundalini   Dormant force, said to be situated at the base of the susumna nadi, which lies along the spine.

Mantra   A sound used for concentration.

Mudra   A seal.

Nadi   A pathway or channel in the subtle body.

Nirguna   Without seed.

Niyama   Personal discipline. The second of Patanjali's eight limbs.

Patanjali   The writer of the *Yoga Sutras*.

Pingala   The nadi or channel that carries the solar energy in the subtle body.

Prakrti   Matter. (The separation of Prakrti and Purusha causes the fluctuation of the gunas.)

Prana   Life force. The breath is an aspect of this.

Pranayama   Regulated breathing which controls Prana. The fourth of Patanjal's eight limbs.

Pratyahara   Withdrawing the senses. The fifth of the eight limbs.

Purusha   Spirit. (The separation of Prakrti and Purusha causes the fluctuation of the gunas.)

Raja Yoga   Usually refers to Patanjali's Yoga system.

Rajas   Activity. One of the three Gunas (tendencies).

Saguna   With seed.

Samadhi   Illumination. The supraconscious state that is the last of Patanjali's eight limbs.

Santosa   Contentment. One of Patanjali's Niyamas.

Sattva   Clarity. One of the three Gunas.

Satya   Truth. One of Patanjali's Yamas.

Saucha   Purity. One of Patanjali's Niyamas.

Siddhis   Supranormal powers.

Susumna   The central nadi (channel) that lies along the spine in the subtle body.

Sutra   A thread. Also teaching given in short aphorisims strung together.

Svadyaya   Study. One of Patanjali's Niyamas.

Tamas   Inertia. One of the three Gunas (tendencies).

Tantra   Extension of Understanding. A religious and cultural movement prominent around AD 1000.

Tapas   Austerity: purificatory action. One of Patanjali's Niyamas.

Turiya   Super conscious state.

Upanishads   Name given to the later Vedas. Literally means 'sitting next to'. Sacred teachings.

Vedas   Sacred hymns and teachings.

Vratyas   Wandering holy men.

Yama   Universal moral commandments. The first of Patanjali's eight limbs.

Yantra   A geometric pattern used as focus for concentration.

Yogi or Yogin   Male practitioner of Yoga.

Yogini   Female practioner of Yoga.

index

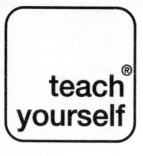

Afrikaans
Access 2002
Accounting, Basic
Alexander Technique
Algebra
Arabic
Arabic Script, Beginner's
Aromatherapy
Astronomy
Bach Flower Remedies
Bengali
Better Chess
Better Handwriting
Biology
Body Language
Book Keeping
Book Keeping & Accounting
Brazilian Portuguese
Bridge
Buddhism
Buddhism, 101 Key Ideas
Bulgarian
Business Studies
Business Studies, 101 Key Ideas
C++
Calculus
Calligraphy
Cantonese
Card Games
Catalan
Chemistry, 101 Key Ideas
Chess
Chi Kung
Chinese
Chinese, Beginner's

Chinese Language, Life & Culture
Chinese Script, Beginner's
Christianity
Classical Music
Copywriting
Counselling
Creative Writing
Crime Fiction
Croatian
Crystal Healing
Czech
Danish
Desktop Publishing
Digital Photography
Digital Video & PC Editing
Drawing
Dream Interpretation
Dutch
Dutch, Beginner's
Dutch Dictionary
Dutch Grammar
Eastern Philosophy
ECDL
E-Commerce
Economics, 101 Key Ideas
Electronics
English, American (EFL)
English as a Foreign Language
English, Correct
English Grammar
English Grammar (EFL)
English, Instant, for French Speakers
English, Instant, for German Speakers
English, Instant, for Italian Speakers
English, Instant, for Spanish Speakers

English for International Business
English Language, Life & Culture
English Verbs
English Vocabulary
Ethics
Excel 2002
Feng Shui
Film Making
Film Studies
Finance for non-Financial Managers
Finnish
Flexible Working
Flower Arranging
French
French, Beginner's
French Grammar
French Grammar, Quick Fix
French, Instant
French, Improve your
French Language, Life & Culture
French Starter Kit
French Verbs
French Vocabulary
Gaelic
Gaelic Dictionary
Gardening
Genetics
Geology
German
German, Beginner's
German Grammar
German Grammar, Quick Fix
German, Instant
German, Improve your
German Language, Life & Culture
German Verbs
German Vocabulary
Go
Golf
Greek
Greek, Ancient
Greek, Beginner's
Greek, Instant
Greek, New Testament
Greek Script, Beginner's
Guitar
Gulf Arabic
Hand Reflexology
Hebrew, Biblical
Herbal Medicine
Hieroglyphics
Hindi
Hindi, Beginner's
Hindi Script, Beginner's

Hinduism
History, 101 Key Ideas
How to Win at Horse Racing
How to Win at Poker
HTML Publishing on the WWW
Human Anatomy & Physiology
Hungarian
Icelandic
Indian Head Massage
Indonesian
Information Technology, 101 Key Ideas
Internet, The
Irish
Islam
Italian
Italian, Beginner's
Italian Grammar
Italian Grammar, Quick Fix
Italian, Instant
Italian, Improve your
Italian Language, Life & Culture
Italian Verbs
Italian Vocabulary
Japanese
Japanese, Beginner's
Japanese, Instant
Japanese Language, Life & Culture
Japanese Script, Beginner's
Java
Jewellery Making
Judaism
Korean
Latin
Latin American Spanish
Latin, Beginner's
Latin Dictionary
Latin Grammar
Letter Writing Skills
Linguistics
Linguistics, 101 Key Ideas
Literature, 101 Key Ideas
Mahjong
Managing Stress
Marketing
Massage
Mathematics
Mathematics, Basic
Media Studies
Meditation
Mosaics
Music Theory
Needlecraft
Negotiating
Nepali

Norwegian
Origami
Panjabi
Persian, Modern
Philosophy
Philosophy of Mind
Philosophy of Religion
Philosophy of Science
Philosophy, 101 Key Ideas
Photography
Photoshop
Physics
Piano
Planets
Planning Your Wedding
Polish
Politics
Portuguese
Portuguese, Beginner's
Portuguese Grammar
Portuguese, Instant
Portuguese Language, Life & Culture
Postmodernism
Pottery
Powerpoint 2002
Presenting for Professionals
Project Management
Psychology
Psychology, 101 Key Ideas
Psychology, Applied
Quark Xpress
Quilting
Recruitment
Reflexology
Reiki
Relaxation
Retaining Staff
Romanian
Russian
Russian, Beginner's
Russian Grammar
Russian, Instant
Russian Language, Life & Culture
Russian Script, Beginner's
Sanskrit
Screenwriting
Serbian
Setting up a Small Business
Shorthand, Pitman 2000
Sikhism
Spanish
Spanish, Beginner's
Spanish Grammar
Spanish Grammar, Quick Fix

Spanish, Instant
Spanish, Improve your
Spanish Language, Life & Culture
Spanish Starter Kit
Spanish Verbs
Spanish Vocabulary
Speaking on Special Occasions
Speed Reading
Statistical Research
Statistics
Swahili
Swahili Dictionary
Swedish
Tagalog
Tai Chi
Tantric Sex
Teaching English as a Foreign Language
Teaching English One to One
Teams and Team-Working
Thai
Time Management
Tracing your Family History
Travel Writing
Trigonometry
Turkish
Turkish, Beginner's
Typing
Ukrainian
Urdu
Urdu Script, Beginner's
Vietnamese
Volcanoes
Watercolour Painting
Weight Control through Diet and Exercise
Welsh
Welsh Dictionary
Welsh Language, Life & Culture
Wills and Probate
Wine Tasting
Winning at Job Interviews
Word 2002
World Faiths
Writing a Novel
Writing for Children
Writing Poetry
Xhosa
Yoga
Zen
Zulu

available from bookshops and on-line retailers

| teach yourself | **relaxation**
richard craze |

- Do you want to learn how to unwind?
- Are you confused by the wealth of relaxation techniques?
- Do you want to find the method that will work for you?

Relaxation explains the techniques of physical and mental relaxation, using disciplines such as meditation, yoga, Alexander Technique, self-hypnosis, affirmations, sleep theraphy, bio-feedback, autogenic training, muscle relaxation, posture exercises and breathing. Choose the method which suits you and bring balance to your life!

Richard Craze is a freelance writer specialising in books on alternative health, new age, religion and other esoteric subjects.

teach
yourself

managing stress
terry looker & olga gregson

- Do you want to understand the theory behind managing stress?
- Do you want to identify the sources of stress in your life?
- Are you looking for you own stress management plan?

Managing Stress is a step-by-step guide to dealing with stress, leading to a healthier, more relaxed and enjoyable way of life. The questionnaire to assess your stress levels will enable you to identify the signs, symptoms and sources of stress. You will understand what is happening to you mentally and physically and you will learn coping strategies to bring balance to your life.

Professor Terry Looker and **Dr Olga Gregson** are Fellows of the international Stress Management Association. They lecture at the Manchester Metropolitan University and worldwide and present stress management programme for industry and the professions.